MEDICAL MASTERCLASS

Clinical Skills

Disclaimer

Although every effort has been made to ensure that drug doses and other information are presented accurately in this publication, the ultimate responsibility rests with the prescribing physician. Neither the publishers nor the authors can be held responsible for any consequences arising from the use of information contained herein. Any product mentioned in this publication should be used in accordance with the prescribing information prepared by the manufacturers.

The information presented in this publication reflects the opinions of its contributors and should not be taken to represent the policy and views of the Royal College of Physicians of London, unless this is specifically stated.

Every effort has been made by the contributors to contact holders of copyright to obtain permission to reproduce copyright material. However, if any have been inadvertently overlooked, the publisher will be pleased to make the necessary arrangements at the first opportunity.

Medical Masterclass

EDITOR-IN-CHIEF

John D. Firth DM FRCP
Consultant Physician and Nephrologist
Addenbrooke's Hospital,
Cambridge

Clinical Skills

EDITORS

John D. Firth DM FRCP
Consultant Physician and Nephrologist
Addenbrooke's Hospital
Cambridge

Claire G. Nicholl MBBS BSc DGM FRCP
Consultant Physician
Department of Medicine for the Elderly
Addenbrooke's Hospital
Cambridge

G. Nicola Rudd MBChB FRCP
Consultant Physician
Palliative Care Team
Leicester Royal Infirmary
Leicester

K. Jane Wilson MBBS MRCP
Consultant Physician
Department of Medicine for the Elderly
Addenbrooke's Hospital
Cambridge

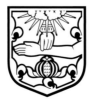

Royal College
of Physicians

© 2004 Royal College of Physicians of London

First published 2001 Blackwell Science Ltd
Reprinted 2004 Royal College of Physicians of London

Published by:
Royal College of Physicians of London
11 St. Andrews Place
Regent's Park
London NW1 4LE
United Kingdom

Set and printed by Graphicraft Limited, Hong Kong

ISBN: 1-86016-217-7 (this book)
ISBN: 1-86016-210-X (set)

Distribution Information:
Jerwood Medical Education Resource Centre
Royal College of Physicians of London
11 St. Andrews Place
Regent's Park
London NW1 4LE
United Kingdom
Tel: 0044 (0)207 935 1174 ext 422/490
Fax: 0044 (0)207 486 6653
Email: merc@rcplondon.ac.uk
Web: http://www.rcplondon.ac.uk/

Contents

List of contributors

John D. Firth DM FRCP
Consultant Physician and Nephrologist
Addenbrooke's Hospital
Cambridge

Debra King MB ChB FRCP
Consultant Physician
Department of Medicine for the Elderly
Wirral Hospital
Wirral
Merseyside

Claire G. Nicholl MBBS BSc DGM FRCP
Consultant Physician
Department of Medicine for the Elderly
Addenbrooke's Hospital
Cambridge

G. Nicola Rudd MBChB FRCP
Consultant Physician
Palliative Care Team
Leicester Royal Infirmary
Leicester

K. Jane Wilson MBBS MRCP
Consultant Physician
Department of Medicine for the Elderly
Addenbrooke's Hospital
Cambridge

Foreword

Since its foundation in 1518, the Royal College of Physicians has engaged in a wide range of activities dedicated to its overall aim of upholding and improving standards of medical practice. *Medical Masterclass* is one of the most innovative and ambitious educational resources the College has developed, and while it continues the tradition of pioneering and supporting high quality medicine, it also makes use of modern day technology by offering computer-assisted learning.

The MRCP(UK) examination is crucial to the progress of physicians through their training. Preparation is not only essential for success in the examination, but it is also important for the acquisition of requisite knowledge, skills and attitudes appropriate for further training. With a pass rate of about 40% at each sitting of the written papers, the exam is a challenge. The College wishes to encourage excellence, and with this in mind has produced *Medical Masterclass*, a comprehensive distance-learning package designed to help candidates with the preparation that is key to making the grade.

Medical Masterclass has been produced by the RCP's Education Department. It represents a formidable amount of work by Dr John Firth and his team of authors and editors. I congratulate our colleagues for this superb educational product and wholeheartedly recommend it as an invaluable MRCP(UK) study aid.

Professor Carol M. Black CBE
President of the Royal College of Physicians

Preface

Medical Masterclass comprises twelve paper-based modules, two CD-ROMs and a companion website. Its aim is to help doctors in their first few years of training to improve their medical skills and knowledge.

The twelve paper-based modules are divided as follows: two cover the scientific background to medicine, one is devoted to general clinical issues, one to emergency medicine and practical procedures, and eight cover the range of medical specialities. Medicine is often fairly straightforward when the diagnosis is clear, but patients rarely come to their doctor and say 'I've got Hodgkin's disease': they have lumps. The core material of each of the clinical specialities is defined by case presentations in the first part of each module: how do you approach the man who has lumps? Structured concise notes on specific diseases follow later. All practising doctors know that medicine is much more than knowing lots of facts about diseases: how do you tell someone they've got cancer? How do you decide when to stop treatment? Most medical texts say little about these issues: *Medical Masterclass* does not avoid them, nor does it talk in vague and abstract terms.

The two CD-ROMs each contain 30 interactive cases requiring diagnosis and treatment. The format is remarkably close to real life: you see the patient and are told the story; you have to decide how to investigate and treat; but you can't see all the results before you start to make decisions!

The companion website, which will be regularly updated, includes self-assessment questions and mock MRCP(UK) exam papers. How much do you know, and are you improving? You will see how your score compares with your previous attempts, and also how your performance compares with others who have logged on to the site.

The *Medical Masterclass* is produced by the Education Department of the Royal College of Physicians. It has been specifically designed to support candidates studying for the MRCP(UK) Examination (All Parts). I have no doubt that someone putting effort into learning through the *Medical Masterclass* would be in a strong position to impress the examiners.

John Firth
Editor-in-Chief

Acknowledgements

Medical Masterclass has been produced by a team. The names of those who have written and edited material are clearly indicated elsewhere, but without the efforts of many other people *Medical Masterclass* would not exist at all. These include Professor Lesley Rees and Mrs Winnie Wade from the Education Department of the Royal College of Physicians of London, who initiated the project; Dr Mike Stein and Dr Andy Robinson from Medschool.com and Blackwell Science respectively, who have enthusiastically supported it from the beginning; and Ms Filipa Maia and Ms Katherine Bowker, who have run the office with splendid efficiency and induced authors and editors to perform to a schedule rarely achieved. I and the whole of the team of editors and authors are immensely grateful to all of these people for the energy that they have poured into *Medical Masterclass* in various ways.

John Firth
Editor-in-Chief

Key features

We have created a range of icon boxes to help you identify key information and to make learning easier and more enjoyable. Here is a brief explanation:

Clinical pointer

This icon highlights important information to be noted.

Further information

This icon indicates the source of further information and reference.

Hints

This icon highlights useful hints, tips and mnemonics.

Key points

This icon is used to highlight points of particular importance.

Quote

This icon indicates useful or interesting citations from notable individuals, including well-known physicians.

Think about

This icon indicates what the reader should reflect on after having read a passage from the text.

Warning/Hazard

This icon is used to indicate common or important drug interactions, pitfalls of practical procedures, or when to take symptoms or signs particularly seriously.

General Clinical Issues

AUTHOR:
J.D. Firth

EDITOR:
G.N. Rudd

EDITOR-IN-CHIEF:
J.D. Firth

The importance of general clinical issues

General clinical issues are those things that are common to the practice of all doctors. They certainly include communication skills, ethical considerations and matters concerned with the accountability of doctors and hospitals to the public. They should also include those aspects of biomedical science that fundamentally underpin clinical practice.

Pieces entitled 'general clinical issues', 'communication skills' or 'medical ethics' are rarely read by doctors and many neglect to even try to keep up to date with biomedical advances. Widespread amongst practising physicians are beliefs that:
• those who write about 'general clinical issues' must be too old and hopeless to write about specific things (which might be of some use)
• those who deal in 'communication skills' don't know any medicine or haven't been near a patient for years (if ever)
• those who talk about 'medical ethics' do not do so in plain English and have never seen a poor old sod who obviously needed to be allowed and helped to die comfortably
• those who make and publish on biomedical advances, be they in molecular biology or meta-analysis, cannot produce anything of relevance to the patients they don't see
• those who deal with the management and organization of health services know nothing about looking after patients.

Some of these beliefs may be justified some of the time, but by no means always, and it is arrogant and wrong for any doctor to think that they could not become a better doctor by learning more about these issues.

Medical Masterclass and 'general clinical issues'

Best medical practice is never from a narrow perspective.

It is not possible to separate the 'communication' or the 'ethics' from the 'medicine'.

In the preface to *The Doctor's Dilemma*, George Bernard Shaw wrote in 1906 that 'wise men used to take care to consult doctors qualified before 1860, who were usually contemptuous of or indifferent to the germ theory ... but now ... we are left in the hands of the generations which ... suddenly concluded that the whole art of healing could be summed up in the formula: find the microbe and kill it'. Why did he write this? There could be many reasons, but the underlying point would seem to be a belief that it was wrong for one specific issue, in this case the germ theory, to dominate all others.

The role of infectious agents in the panoply of diseases is now securely established; but things do change—new pathogens continue to be discovered, as do new roles for known pathogens. Whilst we cannot commend those doctors who were 'contemptuous of or indifferent to the germ theory', most would agree that it would be wrong to argue that the doctor who knew everything about germs knew everything about medicine and healing.

Advances in medicine do not occur across a broad front. The usual analogy is of an amoeba with various pseudopodia—some advancing, some retracting, some becoming very elongated and some disappearing altogether. The whole gradually edges forward, those at the front of the longest pseudopodium often distressed by the lamentable lack of progress. In 1906 the germ experts were in this position: now we would argue that their contribution to medicine is seen in reasonable proportion.

What would Shaw write for the year 2001 and beyond? Three versions that he might consider would be as follows:
• wise men avoid doctors who are experts in 'communication skills', 'ethics' or 'management', but know little medicine
• wise men avoid doctors who behave as if they think that the best practice of medicine can be summed up in the words 'find the gene and clone it'
• wise men avoid doctors who behave as if they think that the best practice of medicine can be summed up in the words 'what are the results of the meta-analysis?'.

How would we respond to these comments? Expertise in communication skills, management, molecular medicine and meta-analysis each have a vast amount to contribute to the present practice and future of medicine, and these topics are rightly discussed in the *Medical Masterclass*. But these valuable techniques should be seen in perspective and used appropriately: they should not be regarded as defining all that is worthwhile in the practice of medicine. Best medical practice is never from a narrow perspective.

Good doctors must know a formidable number of 'medical facts' and make considered judgements based upon them. But this is not enough: they need to be experts in the art of

3

talking to and handling people—people who are sometimes frightened, distressed or angry—and in getting considered judgements across to them in ways that are effective. This is not easy: challenging and rewarding activities never are. There is no single 'right' way of doing things any more than there is a particular hair style that suits everyone best, but there are ways (as hair styles) that are wrong.

Since it is not possible to separate the 'communication' or the 'ethics' from the 'medicine', cases where the main issues are those of communication or ethical decision-making will be discussed in most, if not all, of the clinical modules of the *Medical Masterclass*. In this section entitled 'General Clinical Issues', pains will be taken to avoid vague and vacuous statements, whilst stimulating thought and giving (hopefully) one or two useful tricks of the trade to those who haven't already decided that they can't be bothered to read any further, because it's bound to be boring, tedious and irrelevant.

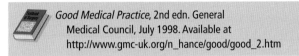

Good Medical Practice, 2nd edn. General Medical Council, July 1998. Available at http://www.gmc-uk.org/n_hance/good/good_2.htm

2 History and examination

The practice of medicine begins with the history and examination.

Requirement for privacy

The history and examination should be conducted in as much privacy as possible. In busy medical admissions units and wards conditions are often 'suboptimal' (ludicrously overcrowded). Some parts of the history and examination cannot be performed in these circumstances and must be deferred to a later time, but not forgotten.

Allow the patient to talk

In 3 minutes, some patients will:
• volunteer a lucid account of their symptoms from the beginning
• specify precisely what their problems are now, contrasting this with their previous state of health
• say what treatments they are taking now, and have taken in the past
• give a concise statement of their past medical history
• mention relevant risk factors for disease, including family history
• state problems or lack of them in other areas
• finish with a succinct summary.

Most patients do not do this but, after taking a history, the doctor should be able to do so on their behalf.

It is not always easy to take a history: some patients won't talk at all and it's impossible to get others to stop, even though it seems increasingly likely that the account of troubles with the grandson, and the stress that this has caused to the daughter (who has bad nerves anyway, which run in the family), has little bearing on the fact that the elderly woman fell down and broke her hip.

When someone suggested to Gary Player that he was lucky to hole a particular golf shot, he is said to have replied, 'the more I practise, the luckier I get'. It is the same with taking a medical history and constructing a differential diagnosis.

 • Allow every patient 3 minutes to tell their story in their own words.
• Speak in a manner that will be understood.
• If you don't understand something, imply that the problem is yours.

Introduce yourself. Say something like 'what's the problem?' and let the patient talk freely, making encouraging noises if necessary to keep them going. If after 3 minutes everything is falling into place, keep quiet and let the patient continue. If it isn't, then you need to intervene.

Say something like 'can we just stop for a minute to make sure that I understand things properly?' This is more generous than saying something which implies, 'you are rambling on in an incoherent manner', since it suggests that the difficulty is yours and not the patient's.

It is standard practice to omit expletives, but you should speak to the patient using comparable language to that which they use. After about a month on a rugby tour with the British Lions, Gareth Edwards (probably the greatest of all scrum halves) asked a fellow player why he had not yet joined in on any conversations, to be told something along the lines, 'I can't keep up with you university types—always using long words like corrugated and marmalade'. There is no point in using words that the patient cannot understand.

• Say: 'you've mentioned a number of things. I just want to be sure I've got the main problem right. What is the main problem?'
• If that doesn't work, try: 'if I could make just one thing better, what would it be?'
• Once you've found out about the main problem, say: 'now what is the next biggest problem?'
• Keep the patient focused on that. Then move on to: 'we've now dealt with the breathing and chest pain, is there anything else?'

No one, in my book, is allowed to have more than three main problems.

Is the patient a reliable witness?

 Not everyone can give a reliable history. If you cannot get a history from the patient, then:
• your notes must explain why
• you must try to get a history from someone else.

Confusion and dementia

It often becomes apparent in the first 30 seconds of conversation that the patient is not a reliable witness. There is no point in taking a lengthy history in this circumstance: it's a waste of time and you can spend your time more profitably doing other things. It is, however, important to document the main concerns that the patient does express: 'my dog, I'm worried that no-one is looking after him', together with evidence of the patient's cognitive state.

Details of the commonly used abbreviated mental test examinations are to be found in *Medicine for the elderly*, Section 3.3, but as an absolute minimum you should record orientation in time, place and person, stating the precise answers that the patient gave: '1938, no; 1940, no'.

The patient should then be asked a few general questions to which they might be able to give a useful answer … 'have you got any pain anywhere?' … but there is no point in trying to drag complex details from someone who doesn't know where they are. The time that you save by not taking a lengthy history from the patient should be spent obtaining information from others: relatives, friends, carers, general practitioners, etc.

Violence, intoxication and madness

A conventional medical history and examination cannot be obtained from someone who is shouting obscenities and breaking up the furniture. The medical notes should describe the situation. Record what you say, verbatim, and the patient's reply, verbatim: this releases tension, and gives an accurate account of the problem if the notes come under scrutiny. The terms 'difficult historian' or 'patient unco-operative' are often seen, but fail to do justice to a drunken axeman. The best medical notes should comment on whether the blows seem to be aimed accurately.

Rare patients will give accounts that are implausible. Take the precaution of giving everyone the benefit of the doubt at first, but if you suspect that the patient is being economical with the truth, obtain details that can be corroborated by others and obtain that corroboration before launching into extensive investigations or acceding to requests or demands for particular treatments. Remain calm under fire: make sure that the patient is not dangerously ill, answer questions simply ('I don't think you need a …'), don't get pushed around and say that it is essential that you get background information.

Asking open questions

 You are likely to get the answers that you ask for.

It is likely that you will be misled if you only ask questions that force particular answers. Ask questions that are open (i.e. do not force or assume particular answers) at least to begin with. For example:
- 'how are you?'
- 'what's the problem?'
- 'when did it start?'
- 'have you any pain?'
- 'have you any difficulty breathing?'
- 'please tell me more about that'.

Immediate formulation of differential diagnosis

 Think about the diagnosis from the beginning, not at the end.

Reading some books and listening to some doctors talk, it is possible to think that the practice of medicine involves taking the history, then performing the examination, then organizing some tests, then reviewing the results, then making the diagnosis, then giving the treatment. This is complete and utter nonsense.

From the moment that you hear of the patient you should be thinking about the diagnosis. For example, a 55-year-old man is coming in with chest pain. As soon as you see the patient, you refine your differential: 'he looks pretty ill to me'. As soon as he opens his mouth, you are refining it further: 'it came on suddenly'.

Directed questions

 Go for the main problem.

After the introductory 'what's the main problem?', the history should not become a multiple choice examination, with all patients set the same paper. Chest pain—yes/no. Breathing problems—yes/no. Orthopnoea—yes/no, etc., etc. I am waiting for someone to object to this: 'surely it's unfair that different patients are asked different questions?'

 When asked why he robbed banks, a criminal replied, 'because that's where the money is'. History taking is the same: focus on the main problem and always keep in mind the list diagnoses that are possible.

After the introductory and open questions, ask directed questions to tease the likely diagnoses in the particular case from as many angles as you are able [1]. For instance, when talking to a man presenting with chest pain, you will ask 'do you suffer from indigestion?' If he says 'no', do not write 'no indigestion' in the notes and leave the topic. Ask:

- 'you've never been troubled at all by it in the past?'
- 'you don't have to take Rennies or anything like that?'
- 'you've never had a barium meal or an endoscopy test in the past?'

Patients rarely try to deliberately mislead the doctor, but they often don't provide the critical information at the first time of asking. It is amazing how many people say 'no' in reply to 'do you suffer from indigestion?', but then admit to taking Rennies regularly and having had a barium meal ('which showed an ulcer') a 'few years ago'.

Helping patients to avoid assumptions

 Get the patient to tell you their symptoms, not their diagnoses.

Some patients persist in giving you their diagnosis of their condition and won't tell you what their symptoms are:

Patient: 'It's indigestion'
Doctor: 'Tell me about the pain'
Patient: 'You know, it's like indigestion'.

After a loop or two of this interaction, the patient then looks at the doctor with the expression 'this doctor's a blithering idiot, they don't even know what indigestion is!' Say:

- 'I know the pain is like indigestion … there are different sorts of indigestion …'
- 'point to where the pain is worst …' (anything to avoid speech and repetition of the dreaded word)
- 'does it go anywhere else?'

Hopefully the ball is now rolling and you can go on to get a description of the symptom to enable you to establish your differential diagnosis.

Importance of the particular and avoidance of the general

 Take a precise history: vague statements are of little value.

At the end of the Olympic 100-metre final, all participants are breathless but the winner is likely to have covered the distance in a shade under 9.9 seconds. Questions such as 'do you ever get breathless?' are totally useless without qualification. If breathing is the problem, ask:

- 'how far can you walk before your breathing stops you?'
- 'did you have to stop when walking from the car park to the clinic?'
- 'when did you last get out of the house?'

It is also critical to establish the patient's 'baseline' condition.

- 'Three months ago, how far could you walk?'

Ask the inpatient who looks blue and breathless:

- 'how does this compare to normal?'
- 'if your breathing was like this at home would you be calling the doctor?'

It is amazing how many say that they wouldn't, and that 'today's quite a good day for them'.

 Note the precise nature of the history elicited by a famous physician in this case:

Christopher Robin had wheezles and sneezles,
They bundled him into his bed.
They gave him what goes with a cold in the nose,
And some more for a cold in the head.
…
They sent for some doctors in sneezles and wheezles
To tell them what ought to be done.
All sorts and conditions of famous physicians
Came hurrying round at a run.
They all made a note of the state of his throat,
They asked if he suffered from thirst;
They asked if the sneezles came *after* the wheezles,
Or if the first sneeze came first …

(A.A. Milne)

Drug history

This is clearly an important aspect of the history of every patient, and for more reasons than might be immediately obvious. The patient's list of drugs or bag of pill bottles is invaluable, as:

- a prompt for history taking: 'why are you on these warfarin pills?' leads to 'oh, I'd forgotten about those … I was given them when I had a clot on my lung …'
- an indication of diagnoses made by previous doctors— but always make sure that the pills were prescribed for the patient; many people take tablets given to other people 'because they helped her, and we thought this was the same sort of thing as she had'.

Family/genetic issues

- Some diagnoses have important implications for other members of the family as well as for the patient.
- Difficult conflicts of interest can arise, for example when performing a test on a patient has serious implications for other family members—such cases are best discussed with a clinical geneticist.

7

All patients should be asked:
- 'are there any diseases or illnesses that run in the family?'
- 'do (or did) your mother and father have any serious medical problems?'
- 'do your brothers or sisters have any serious medical problems?'

If it looks as though the patient might have an uncommon genetic syndrome, ask:
- 'are (or were) your parents related?'
- 'were they cousins?'

Autosomal recessive conditions are much commoner with consanguinity.

Case study of Marfan syndrome

CASE HISTORY

A tall, thin 38-year-old man is admitted as an emergency with chest pain and circulatory collapse. He looks as though he is about to die. The admitting SHO makes the diagnoses of aortic dissection and Marfan syndrome, organizes an urgent CT scan of the chest and refers to the cardiothoracic surgeons whilst this is being done. The patient is taken directly from the scan room to theatre where his ascending aorta is repaired. He recovers well and leaves hospital 10 days later. The SHO presents the case at the main hospital staff round and is congratulated on making the diagnosis and on his management of the case.

Five months later the patient's 36-year-old brother dies suddenly of aortic rupture.

CLINICAL APPROACH

The management of the patient was excellent and rightly applauded. However, the diagnosis of Marfan syndrome had implications not just for the patient, but also for other members of his family. All doctors involved in the patient's care knew that Marfan syndrome was autosomal dominant, with any sibling potentially at 50% risk, but no one had acted on the basis of this knowledge.

The patient's family were contacted and subsequently seen in the clinical genetics clinic: his mother and one surviving brother did not have Marfan syndrome; his father had died suddenly at the age of 45 years, but the family did not know why and did not know any other members of his family; the sister (29 years) did have Marfan syndrome and a slightly dilated aortic root. She was prescribed a β-blocker and arrangements were made for her to be followed annually with echocardiography in the cardiac clinic, with the intention that she should be offered elective surgery if her aorta dilated progressively. She was counselled regarding the risks of pregnancy and childbirth, and also told that any child that she had would be at 50%

risk of having Marfan syndrome. His brother was reassured that he could not pass the condition on to his children.

'Sensitive' issues

- Tackle these last.
- Plan what you are going to say.
- Explain why you want information before you ask for it.

Privacy is important—sensitive questions are less likely to be answered frankly if they are posed in a situation where every comment can be heard by a dozen others.

You must always respect and protect confidential information: but this is particularly important regarding 'sensitive' issues [2].

Some issues are sensitive, including viral (and other) infections associated with particular behaviours, alcohol/drug abuse, psychiatric illness and intimate examinations. These should be left until the end of the history and perhaps until after the examination.
- If a middle-aged man looks jaundiced and has obvious stigmata of chronic liver disease, you should not immediately launch into an inquisition regarding risk factors for cirrhosis.
- If a young man has lost weight, has fevers and a sore mouth due to candida then a likely diagnosis is HIV infection, but to embark immediately on this subject—unless obviously invited to by the patient—would be wrong.
- If an elderly man, recently bereaved, has gone off his food and lost weight, then depression is likely—but you should not jump to this conclusion without a proper history, physical examination and simple tests to exclude other causes.

You do need answers, but you stand a better chance of getting them if you don't dive in.

Case study of chronic liver disease

CASE HISTORY

A middle-aged man is jaundiced and has obvious stigmata of chronic liver disease. You need to ask him about risk factors.

CLINICAL APPROACH

Obtain all other details of the history first. Hopefully you will gain the trust and confidence of the patient: 'this doctor's trying to help me'. Then introduce the questions

that you are about to ask, don't just blurt them out. Say to the patient:
- 'there is obviously a problem with your liver ...'
- 'I need to ask some questions about things that can cause liver disease ...' (the patient may volunteer information)
- 'liver disease can be caused by alcohol or by some viruses ...' (patient may volunteer information)
- 'have you ever been a heavy drinker? ...' (patient may volunteer information)
- 'you've never been a 10 pint a day man ... or a bottle of spirits a day man? ...' (patient may volunteer information)
- 'are you at risk of viral infection? ...' (patient may volunteer information)
- 'the commonest viruses that can cause liver disease are hepatitis B and hepatitis C ...' (patient may volunteer information)
- 'the risk factors for these are blood transfusions, intravenous drug use with shared needles, homosexual relationships ...' (patient may volunteer information)
- 'have you had any ... ? etc., etc.'

It is my firm impression that an approach such as this gives the best chance of obtaining the necessary information.

Many doctors find themselves embarrassed by some of the questions necessary to obtain a complete history when diseases such as hepatitis B or HIV infection are possible or proven. Indeed, the questions are not those that the doctor is likely to ask, or the patient to answer, in any context other than the medical consultation. This is the key: with explanation of the reason for the doctor wanting to ask the question, patients will not be mortally offended and will provide answers. If the doctor becomes awkward half way through, then the whole thing can begin to seem improper and an embarrassing situation can arise. Remember a form of words that suits you, adopt a professional and formal manner and press on.

Case study of rectal examination

CASE HISTORY

An elderly man has lost weight. You need to perform a rectal examination, and he looks very surprised when you suggest this.

CLINICAL APPROACH

If patients present to their doctor with a bowel or urinary problem, they will generally not be surprised if the doctor wants to 'check their tail end' and perform an 'internal examination'. Many patients are surprised if the doctor asks to do this apparently 'out of the blue'. The approach to this problem might be as follows:
- 'you have lost a lot of weight and we need to find out why ...'
- 'sometimes problems in the bowel or pelvis can cause this ...'
- 'I therefore need to examine the back passage ...'
- 'can you pull down your trousers and ... etc.'

If you feel it proper to do so for any reason, arrange for a chaperone before proceeding [3]. Say to the patient: 'I need some help for this'.

Case study of depression

CASE HISTORY

An elderly man, recently bereaved, has lost a great deal of weight and is referred to hospital. There are no other symptoms, examination is unremarkable and screening tests are 'negative'. You think that depression is likely but as soon as you broach the subject he becomes defensive and says 'I'm not depressed'. You are unsure, and would like the patient to see a psychiatrist.

CLINICAL APPROACH

Many patients (and regrettably some doctors) continue to believe that there is something dishonourable about having depression or other psychiatric illnesses. When their symptoms take them to a physician they are often very reluctant to accept that there isn't—as they see it—a 'real' (clear physical) basis for their problems. In this case you could say something along the following lines:
- 'you have lost a lot of weight ...'
- 'there could be many reasons for this ...'
- 'at the start I wondered about a number of conditions, including serious things like cancer ...'
- 'but I'm pleased to say I cannot find any evidence of anything like that ...'
- 'I've examined you thoroughly, and everything seems in reasonable order ...'
- 'the tests have shown nothing terrible ...'
- 'I cannot be absolutely sure, but my honest opinion is that the problem may be that—very understandably after the death of your wife—you have become depressed ...'
- 'I am not saying that you are mad or anything like that ...'
- 'depression can be a natural reaction ... everyone gets depressed to some degree from time to time ... and many people get depressed after the death of a loved one ... indeed, it's a bit odd if they don't ...'
- 'what I would like to suggest is that we get an expert opinion ...'
- 'I would like you to talk to a psychiatric colleague of mine ...'
- 'that's all I would like you to do ... just talk to them ...'
- 'would it be alright for me to arrange this? ...'

• 'they might be able to help us … and if we don't talk to them, we won't know …'.

This line of conversation cannot be guaranteed to work, but it's a straightforward and honest presentation that many will accept. However, if the patient will not accept psychiatric referral, then this cannot be forced upon them unless they are judged to be a risk to themselves or others. See *Psychiatry*, Sections 2.6 and 2.11 for further discussion, and remember to phone this man's general practitioner before he goes home, particularly if he insists on declining psychiatric review.

Differential diagnosis

 Always write down your working differential diagnoses.

You should always finish a clerking by writing down your working differential diagnoses, listed in order of probability. If in doubt, bet on a common diagnosis rather than a rare one and take particular care to make sure that you always consider—even if only briefly and to dismiss—diagnoses that are serious (potentially fatal) and treatable.

Medical notes

 Always write proper notes.

Good notes help doctors who come after you immensely. They provide a succinct summary of the information you gathered at the time, the conclusions that you drew and the actions that followed.

The notes made by many doctors are incredibly bad. If you are not impressed by the thought that they might help (or hinder) your colleagues in sorting out some problem in the future, then remember that they are legal records.

Whilst practising medicine with one eye on what the courts might think has substantial disadvantages for both doctors and patients, if such consideration were to lead to improved note keeping, then this would be a good thing.

Explanation and consent

It is crucial that procedures are explained to patients in terms that they can understand. This is necessary for consent to investigation and treatment, and carries the additional and substantial advantage that the patient is much more likely to be able to put up with something if they know what's going to happen. Being in pain under a green towel with someone stabbing your neck must be particularly alarming if you've no idea how long it's going to go on for or why the doctor is doing it.

Explain why you think that the procedure is required, how the results could help the patient, and be frank and open about what is involved, the risks and the alternatives to the investigation or treatment that you are proposing.

The doctor providing the treatment or undertaking an investigation is responsible for obtaining consent. In many cases this task is delegated, but it can only be performed properly by someone with a sufficient understanding of the procedure or treatment involved [4]. If you are not sure about any of the issues then find out from a senior colleague, or ask such a colleague to talk to the patient. Write what you have told the patient in the notes, especially regarding the risks, and make sure that any consent form required by the hospital is properly completed.

1 Rubenstein D, Wayne D, Bradley JR. The clinical approach. In: *Lecture Notes on Clinical Medicine*, 5th edn. Oxford: Blackwell Science, 1997.

2 The duties of a doctor. In: *Good Medical Practice*. Available at http://www.gmc-uk.org/n_hance/good/doad.htm

3 Intimate examinations are a frequent cause of complaint to the General Medical Council. Available at http://www.gmc-uk.org/n_hance/good/intimate.htm

4 Seeking patients' consent: the ethical considerations. General Medical Council, February 1999. Available at http://www.gmc-uk.org/n_hance/good/consent.htm

Communication skills

Talking to patients

All doctors need to talk to patients at some time or another about good news, uncertainty and bad news.

> ! **Talking about good news, uncertainty and bad news**
>
> Good news:
> - reassure when it is reasonable to do so.
>
> Uncertainty and bad news:
> - be honest
> - explain things slowly, and as fully as you can
> - give explanation to those who want it
> - don't force things onto people who don't want to hear
> - confirm continued care
> - offer to talk to relatives.
>
> Unrealistic expectations:
> - appear sympathetic
> - don't try to do things that can't be done.
>
> Always:
> - offer to answer any questions.
>
> Never:
> - embark on a difficult conversation that you know you don't have time for: make apologies and come back later.

Good news

 To refuse to offer reassurance is bad medicine.

Case study of non-cardiac chest pain

CASE HISTORY

A 58-year-old man has been admitted with chest pain which went away before admission and has not recurred overnight. He is terrified that he might have had a coronary. You cannot make a confident positive diagnosis but nothing supports a diagnosis of ischaemic heart disease. Serial ECGs and cardiac enzymes are normal and the man does not look unwell.

CLINICAL APPROACH

It is always impossible to prove that somebody hasn't got something, but the doctor who refuses to offer reassurance when it is reasonable to do so serves the patient badly.

You could say something like:
- 'I (or we) am not sure what caused your pain …'

- 'the obvious worry was angina or a heart attack, but the pain has not come back and the good news is that all of the tests of the heart are satisfactory …'
- 'there is no evidence you've got angina or had a heart attack …'
- 'it could have been due to indigestion, but I'm not sure about this …'
- 'I don't think you need to stay in hospital now or need any more tests at the moment, etc.'

You would, of course, go on to explain that the patient should report immediately to his doctor if pain recurs; make arrangements for further tests and follow-up if considered appropriate; and arrange for details of admission to be sent promptly to the patient's doctor.

It is always impossible to exclude disease with 100% certainty, but to refuse to offer reassurance is bad medicine.

Uncertainty

Case study of probable lung cancer

CASE HISTORY

A 68-year-old man who smoked heavily for many years is admitted with a chest infection. The appearances on the chest radiograph make it very likely that he has lung cancer.

CLINICAL APPROACH

If you have already talked to the man, you will have gained some impression of his character. If you have not, then you should begin by introducing yourself and talking about his symptoms and problems. Ask him what he thinks is going on. He may volunteer several concerns, including the possibility of cancer, but most likely will say that he thinks he's got a chest infection.

How do you take it from here? I would confirm that he has got a chest infection, but then say something along the lines of:
- 'but there might be something more serious …'
- 'are you the sort of man who likes to know exactly what's going on?'

This prepares the patient for the possibility of bad news without giving the news itself. Most patients say that they want to know what's going on and you can proceed to say that there's some shadowing on the chest radiograph that will need to be looked into further. Most patients will immediately think of cancer and some will ask straight out 'is it cancer?', to which you can reply 'it might be, but I can't be definite without other tests' (usually true). Other patients will not ask any questions and you should confine yourself to saying that 'further tests will be needed'.

The patient may ask 'is it cancer?' the next day: but there is no sense and justification in pressing this news on someone faster than they are prepared to accept it. Indeed, it is cruel to do so and the patient who seems plainly not to want to know should not be force-fed unpalatable information.

Bad news

- Do not give a patient bad news when you don't have any time to talk.
- The patient should be given as much information as they want.
- It is cruel to force information onto someone who clearly doesn't want to know.
- Always reassure that symptoms will be treated.
- Always reassure that the patient will not be 'written off' by the doctors.

When a number of tests are planned or results are awaited, it is useful to arrange to speak to the patient (often with their relatives) to discuss everything together—'can we talk on Thursday afternoon at 3 o'clock when all the test results should be back?' This avoids having multiple unsatisfactory discussions, each culminating in 'we need the result of the next test', and lets the patient know where they stand.

Case study of inoperable lung cancer

CASE HISTORY

A 68-year-old man who smoked heavily for many years is admitted with a chest infection. The infection is slow to clear and sputum cytology and CT scan of the chest confirm inoperable lung cancer.

CLINICAL APPROACH

You need 5 minutes to talk about this sort of thing: don't tackle it when you can only afford 30 seconds. In previous discussions you should have got to know the patient, but if not, then you need to introduce yourself and talk about his problems for a minute or so.

To take matters further, you might say something along the lines:
- 'I know you are the sort of man who likes to know what is going on …'

- 'I am afraid that the test results are not good …' (prepares for bad news, the patient may ask 'is it cancer?')
- 'the tests on your spit and the scan have shown a serious problem …' (more preparation for bad news; the patient may ask 'is it cancer?')
- 'they show that you have got a cancer in the lung'.

Speak slowly, do not hurry, look the man in the face, hold his hand or touch him on the arm if that seems appropriate.

The man may immediately begin to ask questions:
- 'is it curable?'
- 'do I need an operation?'
- 'will I die?'

These should be answered simply and truthfully, but never remove all hope. You cannot be sure how long the man will live for: doctors have been known to get things wrong. If he says 'is it days or weeks?', say 'I don't know … we need to see how things go'.

When appropriate explain that treatment for symptoms is always available. Confirm that things will be done to help as much as is possible. Don't leave the patient with the impression that nothing can be done and the doctors are washing their hands of the problems. Offer to answer any questions, to speak to relatives, and say that you or one of your colleagues will come back again.

Unrealistic expectations

- Some people are unrealistic.
- Search with reasonable diligence for illnesses.
- Do not embark on endless series of investigations.
- Always be sympathetic to those who are frustrated by their limitations.

Some patients have unrealistic expectations of themselves, and some people have unrealistic expectations of their partners. I recently saw a splendidly fit 84-year-old man, referred because of breathlessness and '?cardiac failure'. When we got down to it, the specific complaint was that he was no longer able to play three sets of tennis; the first two were OK, but he struggled in the third. His heart was in splendid shape.

You should always look with reasonable diligence for things that treatment might improve, but should be frank in saying what you can't do.

Always be sympathetic to those who are frustrated by their limitations.

Some doctors embark on a never-ending programme of investigation: if the first series of tests show no substantial abnormality then it is quite probable that something minor will be revealed, or that they will order more. Minor abnormalities then become the focus of further tests, and if enough of these are done, then more minor abnormalities will undoubtedly be forthcoming—'big fleas have smaller fleas on their backs to bite them'.

This is not good medicine: much anxiety is generated, much money is spent and no good is done. You should refrain from initiating interminable series of investigations that have little or no chance of showing anything that might benefit the patient. Say:

- 'I am pleased to be able to tell you everything seems satisfactory ...'
- 'I can find nothing terrible when I examine you ...'
- 'all the tests done have given satisfactory results ...'
- 'the blood tests show that you are not anaemic and the kidney, liver and bone tests do not show anything alarming ...' (covers for very minor abnormalities you may have elected not to pursue)
- 'there is no evidence of inflammation in the blood ...' (you have probably checked the erythrocyte sedimentation rate (ESR) or C-reative protein (CRP) and immunoglobulins)
- 'the chest radiograph and the electrical tracing of your heart are satisfactory ...'
- 'I do not think that any further tests would be helpful'.

Most patients are reassured by this and are grateful that you have taken the time and trouble to check things over so thoroughly. Many feel better simply for knowing that you haven't found anything seriously amiss and will say something along the lines:

- 'I wanted to get things checked over, but ...'
- 'I thought it was probably just that I was getting old'.

However, some patients are unwilling to accept reassurance and may suggest or try to insist on other tests:

- 'shouldn't I have a CT scan of my abdomen?'

If this is warranted in your opinion, then you should organize the investigation after discussion with your radiological colleagues. If you judge that it is not clinically indicated, then you should explain quietly but firmly to the patient why this is so, but not allow yourself to be pressurized into a course of medical action that you feel is unjustified. Offer the patient an opportunity of speaking with your consultant. They may say: 'I want a second opinion'. They are entitled to request this, usually through their general practitioner, but you or your consultant should be willing to provide the names of suitable physicians if this is requested.

Death and dying

Death is anticipated

To put it mildly: this is a problem for almost everyone—the patient, their partner, relatives and friends, carers, nurses and doctors. Rare individuals can comfortably face the prospect of their own death; most struggle in one way or another.

Most are frightened

Aubade

I work all day, and get half-drunk at night.
Waking at four to soundless dark, I stare.
In time the curtain-edges will grow light.
'Til then I see what's really always there:
Unresting death, a whole day nearer now,
Making all thought impossible but how
And where and when I shall myself die.
Arid interrogation: yet the dread
Of dying, and of being dead,
Flashes afresh to hold and horrify.
The mind blanks at the glare. Not in remorse
—The good not done, the love not given, time
Torn off unused—nor wretchedly because
An only life can take so long to climb
Clear of its wrong beginnings, and may never;
But the total emptiness for ever,
The sure extinction that we travel to
And shall be lost in always. Not to be here,
Not to be anywhere,
And soon; nothing more terrible, nothing more true.
This is a special way of being afraid
No trick dispels ...
... Postmen like doctors go from house to house.

(Philip Larkin)

Some are angry

Do Not Go Gentle into that Good Night

Do not go gentle into that good night,
Old age should burn and rave at close of day;
Rage, rage against the dying of the light.
Grave men, near death, who see with blinding sigh
Blind eyes could blaze like meteors and be gay,
Rage, rage against the dying of the light.
And you, my father, there on the sad height,
Curse, bless me now with your fierce tears, I pray.
Do not go gentle into that good night.
Rage, rage against the dying of the light.

(Dylan Thomas)

How should the doctor behave?

Do not race past with eyes down and avoid the patient. Ask them if they would like anything to be done. Talk about their symptoms and offer treatment for them. Offer the opportunity of going home if this is possible. Make it clear that you care and arrange for a cigarette if that's what the patient wants.

See *Pain relief and palliative care*, Section 2.

Do Not Resuscitate orders

> Do Not Resuscitate orders are a medical decision.
>   IF you discuss Do Not Resuscitate orders with a patient, you MUST make it absolutely clear that:
> - you are NOT asking 'do you want to die?'
> - you are NOT asking 'do you want treatment?'.
>   If you are in doubt, then the patient should be for resuscitation.

In many hospitals in the UK it is 'official policy' to discuss Do Not Resuscitate (DNR) orders with patients and their relatives. It is much less common that doctors actually do so, usually because they fear that they will cause distress to people who know they are dying but haven't thought about the moment of death, don't want to do so for obvious reasons, and could be given the impression that the doctor initiating such a conversation was 'writing them off'. Initiating a DNR order without talking to the patient is usually justified on the grounds that such a discussion would not be possible or 'not be in the patient's best interest'. In my view this is entirely correct behaviour in many cases, but sometimes the patient will bring the subject up and sometimes it seems proper for the doctor to do so.

If approached correctly, the subject of 'Do Not Resuscitate' is much easier to talk about than it sounds. You are NOT saying to the patient:
- 'do you want to die … yes or no?' or
- 'do you want us to try to make you better … yes or no?' and you MUST make this absolutely clear.

Case study of disseminated cancer

CASE HISTORY

A 67-year-old woman has disseminated breast cancer. She is admitted with fitting due to cerebral metastases. The fitting stops with benzodiazepines, she is started on dexamethasone and comes round so that she can hold a sensible conversation. The nurse asks you 'is she for resus?'.

CLINICAL APPROACH

If you judge it proper to speak to the patient, do so in the company of the nurse. Begin by introducing yourself and explaining what has happened in simple terms. Even if you have seen the woman before, she may well not remember. Ask her if she wants to know details of what has happened (begin with the past). If, as is likely, she says 'yes', then explain, simply and slowly, what has been done, and what you hope it will achieve (move to the future): '… reduce the swelling in the brain and help stop the fits'.

At this point it is important to find out what the woman understands about her own condition: 'have the doctors you have seen before had a chance to talk to you about what's going on?' (not, 'what do you know about your illness?' or anything else that implies it's an exam and that she will lose marks for not giving a lucid and comprehensive answer).

It is likely that she will know and understand that her days are numbered. It may be that issues such as resuscitation have been discussed with her before, and she may indicate this:
- 'Dr Brown talked about it with me in the clinic …'
- 'I understand the situation …'
- 'I have made a living will …'.

If this is not the case I would then go on to talk about resuscitation and further treatment, probably as follows:
- 'we both know that this problem won't go away …'
- 'if you were to get very ill then I wouldn't want to put you through pain and discomfort …'
- 'I would plan to give simple treatments and make sure that you weren't uncomfortable …' (you are not saying that you won't treat her)
- 'I wouldn't be planning to put tubes in your neck or throat, take you to the intensive care unit, or jump up and down on your chest …'
- 'there wouldn't be any point, they wouldn't help …'
- 'I would want to make sure that you were comfortable and didn't have any pain …' (you will keep looking after the patient and not write them off)
- 'is that alright?'

Most patients will nod or say 'yes'; many will say 'thank you'. If the patient says anything at any time, then stop and listen. Answer questions simply and honestly. Offer to explain things to relatives.

Make an appropriate entry in the medical records and ensure that the nurses know (if one has not been present).

If this patient had not recovered to the point where they could hold a sensible conversation, then it would clearly not be possible to hold any discussion along these lines with her and I would make a decision that she was not for resuscitation, tell the nurse, and make the appropriate entry for the notes. I would justify this decision on the grounds that attempts to resuscitate would be futile, meaning that they could not be expected to prolong meaningful life.

Very rarely, a patient will tell you that they 'want everything done', and may say this despite explanation that aggressive interventions would be futile and could be painful and unpleasant. My approach in this situation would be to agree to 'do everything reasonable', but in practice I would not strive as officiously as I would in other circumstances. Most doctors behave similarly in this uncommon situation.

See *Haematology*, Section 1.7.

Relatives

Relatives come in all shapes and sizes. Many are wonderful; some are not.

'Don't let the patient know'

 In 99% of cases this is the relatives' problem, not the patient's.

Case study of suspected malignancy

CASE HISTORY

A 72-year-old man is admitted with weight loss and vomiting. You suspect malignancy and arrange for upper gastrointestinal endoscopy. His daughter says 'if it's bad news … don't let him know'.

CLINICAL APPROACH

You will already have talked to the patient, and if you have spoken to him along the lines described above, you will know whether he wants to know what's going on and may already have discussed your suspicions with him.

In 99 cases out of 100, the problem here is the daughter's and not the patient's, but it would be unkind and unhelpful to say so. Ask her what she's concerned about. Tell her that you've already spoken to her father about things and recount that conversation. Say that he does know what's going on, and wants to be told.

Most patients want to talk to the doctor about bad news and can do so. Most relatives want to talk to the doctor about bad news and can do so. Many patients and relatives find it extremely difficult to talk to each other about bad news, at least to begin with. After speaking with the daughter I would make a point of taking her to her father, sitting down with them, and briefly repeating what I've said to each to both together. This takes 3 minutes, helps future communication enormously, and saves a great deal of time in the long run.

See *Oncology*, Section 1.9.

Unexpected death of a patient

- You, a nurse and the relative need privacy and somewhere to sit down.
- Give your bleep to someone else for 5 minutes.
- Speak slowly and quietly.
- Don't say too much.
- Don't be afraid of silence and tears.

Case study of sudden death

CASE HISTORY

A 51-year-old business man collapses at work. An emergency ambulance is called and he is brought directly into the medical admissions unit. Your attempts to resuscitate him fail. One of the nurses tells you that his wife has just arrived: 'can you speak to her?'

CLINICAL APPROACH

There is no easy way to do this.
- Find a nurse to accompany you. Make sure that there is a private room available. Give your bleep to someone else if possible.
- Introduce yourself to the patient's wife, say 'we need to talk …' (she will assume bad news).
- Lead her to the private room and get her to sit down; say 'I have some very bad news …' (she may assume the worst).
- Speak slowly and don't say too much … 'when your husband was brought here his heart was very weak … we tried to get it going … but we couldn't'.
- She might answer 'you mean he's dead?'
- Nod your head … 'I'm afraid he is'.
- People do not usually think rationally at this time. You may be asked questions that are relevant or ridiculous. Do not be afraid of silence and tears. Try to answer simply and honestly.
- Reassure the wife that her husband did not suffer: 'he was not aware of what was going on'.
- When appropriate, make your excuse to leave, 'I must go now … I will leave you with the nurse … if you would like to speak to me again, then please let the nurse know'.
- Tell the wife that she can see the body 'as soon as it's ready'. Leave quietly.
- Inform the patient's doctor about what has happened.

Relatives and Do Not Resuscitate orders

 Do Not Resuscitate orders are a medical decision.
- Talk to relatives and discern their views.
- If a patient cannot speak for him or herself, find out (in appropriate circumstances) if they have expressed views in the past or completed a living will.
    BUT
- Do NOT ask relatives to decide, or make them think they are deciding.
- Do NOT imply that relatives have a 'casting vote'.

It may be proper to discuss DNR orders with relatives, but it is always totally improper to ask them to make the decision, or even to imply to them that they have a casting vote in the matter. Few things can make people feel more worried and more guilty for more years, for a less good reason.

Do Not Resuscitate orders are a matter for medical decision-making, in the same way that the decision to use a particular antibiotic is. For choice of antibiotic it is appropriate to listen to the advice of the microbiologist, but the decision remains with the prescribing physician. For DNR orders it is appropriate to listen to the patient, their relatives, and other professionals involved in the patient's care—but the decision remains with the doctors.

It is possible to find out the views of relatives about aggressive medical treatment of the patient without asking direct questions such as 'would you like us to use a breathing machine, etc?' If asked such questions, the relatives might reasonably conclude that they are being asked to make the decision, even if this was not the doctor's intent.

If the patient is unable to speak for him or herself, then—in appropriate situations—it may be possible to find out what their views are likely to be from the relatives. When talking to the daughter of a man with a long history of bad chronic obstructive pulmonary disease, now in extremis, it would be reasonable to say:
• 'did he ever talk about what might happen if his breathing got as bad as this?'
• 'did he ever talk about breathing machines?'

If the answer to these questions is 'no', then there is no point in pursuing this line of discussion, but if the daughter says:
• 'he said he wanted to be allowed to go'
• 'he said he never wanted to have anything to do with them'
• 'he's done one of those living wills'

… then this is helpful information and should be considered in medical decision-making.

If the patient is clearly dying, speak along the following lines:
• 'I don't know how things are going to go over the next few hours and days …'
• 'it may be that he will slip away …' (you are not afraid to mention death, indirectly at first)
• 'and if he is dying, we must make sure that he's comfortable and not in any pain …' (you will not ignore him if he is dying)
• 'there wouldn't be any point in jumping up and down on his chest, it wouldn't do any good and would make him uncomfortable …' (you [the doctors] have made the decision not to attempt resuscitation).

Virtually all relatives will accept this, and many will say 'thank you'. If they say anything, then stop and listen. Answer questions simply and honestly.

Make an appropriate entry in the medical records and ensure that the nurses know (if one has not been present).

Very rarely, a relative will say that they 'want everything done' despite explanation that aggressive interventions would be futile and could be painful and unpleasant. My approach in this situation would be to agree to 'do everything reasonable', but in practice I would not strive as officiously as I would in other circumstances. Most doctors behave similarly in this uncommon situation.

Anger and complaints

 Anger is usually an expression of distress.

• Take a nursing or medical colleague with you when you speak to angry relatives.
• Get everyone to sit down.
• Make sure you are nearest the door.
• Allow the person to say what they want to say.
• Speak softly, simply and honestly.
• Don't get angry yourself.
• Don't take it personally.
• Write full notes.

People respond in a variety of ways to finding that one of their relatives has been admitted to hospital. Many are exceedingly helpful; most make entirely reasonable and appropriate enquiries and comments (which may include reasonable and justified specific complaints); some keep away; some get angry and complain about everything.

Case study of a large stroke

CASE HISTORY

An 81-year-old woman is admitted after a large stroke. She is still on the ward 3 weeks later, having made little recovery. She is severely dysphasic so communication is very difficult; she needs to be fed and given drinks by the nurses and dribbles both down her chin; she slumps to the side in her chair; she is incontinent of urine and has a catheter. Yesterday she fell out of her chair and bruised her cheek; she looks a mess. Whenever her son visits he complains to the nurses (who had told his wife about the injury over the phone when it happened) about everything. Today he is extremely angry, and the nurse in charge of the ward asks you to speak to him.

CLINICAL APPROACH

Do not tackle this sort of problem on your own. Take a nursing or medical colleague with you. Introduce yourself to the patient's son, and then lead the way to a private office on the ward. Sit down, with yourself and your colleague nearest to the door, and say:

- 'I am so sorry that your mother has had this stroke'.
  This sometimes disarms the angry before they start.

If the son immediately launches into a statement, then keep quiet until he appears to have finished. If he says nothing, then begin, with something along the lines:

- 'I wanted to talk to you about things ...' (the doctor does not want to brush anything under the carpet)
- 'your mother came in 3 weeks ago with a big stroke, and I'm afraid that she has not got much better ...' (start off with a simple summary of the problems as you see them)
- 'she cannot speak properly, she cannot eat and drink without help, her balance is poor and she leans to the side ... she slumped out of the chair yesterday and banged the side of her face ...' (the doctor isn't avoiding the problem)
- 'we are trying to help with physiotherapy and exercises, but I'm afraid that there is a limit to what we can do'.

Speak slowly and quietly; look the son in the eye; if he interrupts, then let him say what he wants to. If (when) he says:

- 'she shouldn't have been allowed to fall ...'
- 'the nurses on this ward are no good ...'
- 'I've told them lots of times that she shouldn't be left ...'.

Then let him finish speaking, and say something like:

- 'we are all sorry that she fell ...'
- 'her balance is very bad ...'
- 'she had been carefully propped in the chair (assuming she was) ...'
- 'but unfortunately she fell out ...'
- 'we would like to, but I am afraid that we cannot have a nurse standing by her chair or bed 24 hours a day ...'
- 'we only have three nurses for a ward with 30 beds'.

If the son says he's going to complain, then:

- Say quietly that it is his right to do so.
- Offer to tell him about the correct mechanism for doing so (usually via the hospital's 'patient satisfaction office') in the unlikely event that he doesn't know already.
- Offer him the possibility of an appointment with the consultant.
- Make clear notes in the medical records, stating who was present and what was said—if the son swore at you or the nurses, then write this down verbatim (releases tension, and gives an accurate record of the problem if the notes come under scrutiny).

Do not get angry. These things happen to all doctors, often regarding cases where they and the nurses have tried particularly hard. The relatives who complain the most are often those who have seen the patient least.

 Smith R. A good death: an important aim for health services and for us all. *BMJ* 2000; 320: 129–130.

4 Being a doctor

4.1 Team work and errors

Team work

The main question is: 'how do you get the team on your side?'

Hospitals are complex things and caring for patients is often a complicated business. Lots of people are involved. The vast majority are trying to do a good job, would like to do it even better, but are limited (as are you) by the number of hours in the day, the resources available and processes that aren't necessarily under their control.

When a decision regarding the investigation or management of a patient has been made, the question becomes, 'how can we do this?', or in many cases, 'how do you get other members of the hospital team to do the things that you want?'

Observation of doctors reveals a number of strategies, some subtle and some not: these would include—in alphabetical order, rather than order of frequency or effectiveness—anger, bullying, charm, humour, pleading, seduction, shouting and threats. Some doctors are selective, employing one device in one situation and another in another. Some are not: we have all met those whose response to any problem is to hit it with a hammer, and if that fails they go off to find a bigger hammer.

The bottom line is this: you can have made a brilliant diagnosis or proposed a brilliant treatment, but—such is the requirement for team work in most things in the hospital—if you cannot get others to see things the way that you do and take action that you would like them to, then the patient rarely benefits from your brilliance. All doctors need to be able to work as part of a team, and where appropriate assume the responsibilities of team leader [1].

Errors

- It is uncommon for one person to be totally to blame for any error or accident.
- Giving someone a 'dressing down' in public causes more problems than it solves.
- If you want to let off steam, blame the individual; if you want to sort out problems, fix the systems.

Errors occur in all human endeavours, including medicine. When they are made it is almost always due to a combination of factors, some related to the system and some to the individual. This is known as the 'Swiss cheese' model: if each slice of cheese is a part of the system or an individual in the system, and each hole is a problem or fault in the part of the system or performance of the individual, then when the holes become aligned, a clear path is seen from one side of the block of cheese to the other, and an 'accident' can slip through.

It is uncommon for one person to be totally to blame for any error or accident, and doctors working in teams should always remember this. When problems do arise, issues are best handled at the time with a light touch (but one that gives the impression it could become firmer) and no shouting or obscenities. It is rarely, if ever, helpful to give anyone a 'dressing down' in public, and often immensely unhelpful. This is not to say that errors should be tolerated, simply that 'blaming someone' is rarely an effective solution: the immediate therapeutic benefit of 'letting off steam' is invariably outweighed by the long-term repercussions of having done so.

All organizations that have less than their fair share of accidents expect to make errors and talk about the possibilities [2]. When errors or accidents occur they do not hide them, but discuss them openly and try to develop mechanisms to prevent them from recurring. They encourage every individual to think about what they do and to say when they spot something that could lead to an accident. Is this how your ward, unit or hospital work? If not, then it should be.

Other doctors

Get the reputation—'if Bloggs wants something, there's bound to be a good reason'.

'How do you get other doctors on your side?'

Senior doctors can always try to bully junior ones and unfortunately some do, but this isn't a proper way to behave and is generally a mark of insecurity in the senior doctor, or just plain nastiness. Your colleagues may do things for you because they are frightened of you or because they like you, but it's virtually impossible to be feared by or liked by everyone. The best method is to get yourself into a position where you are respected. This is not to be confused with having an important title in the hospital or medical school. There is an association between important titles and respect, but this association is not as strong as some would believe, and respect attaches to the individual and not to their position.

The following are some characteristics of doctors who are respected by their colleagues, who can therefore get them to do things when they want them to be done:

- They try their best
- They are knowledgeable
- They are not frightened to say 'I don't know'
- They don't hide when the going gets tough
- (They have a dislike of long lists and pious ramblings).

Case study of 'unwell' with abdominal and back pain

1 A man is admitted with vague abdominal and back pain. He looks unwell. The doctor cannot make a confident diagnosis but wonders about the possibility that it is renal colic. He phones the radiologist in the ultrasound department that morning to discuss the case, and the patient has a plain abdominal film and an ultrasound later in the day. This reveals a large abdominal aortic aneurysm.
2 A man is admitted with vague abdominal and back pain. He looks unwell. The doctor cannot make a confident diagnosis but wonders about the possibility that it is due to an abdominal aortic aneurysm. He places an order for an abdominal ultrasound which says 'abdo pain?cause'. This is not done that day.

Who do you think is the better doctor?

Professions allied to medicine

- Show respect for the expertise of other professionals.
- Ask nurses and other colleagues for their views and comments.
- Give praise where praise is due.

Doctors work as part of a team but are in a privileged position, by which I mean that they generally give more orders than they take. Some abuse this position and speak to nursing and other staff in a manner that is appalling, usually when they are tired and when no one else is around. This is always a sign of immaturity, nastiness or both.

Make a deliberate point of asking nurses and other professionals allied to medicine for their views about the patients they are caring for. They will often know a great deal more than you or your medical colleagues do about some things and it is ridiculous not to make use of this information when making decisions.

Things do not always go smoothly; if a ward rings in the middle of the night with a fatuous request (03:00 hours—'can you rewrite one of the drug charts for the morning') then arrange to speak to the ward manager

the next time you are both on duty at the same time. In modern jargon, the 'process' needs to be reconsidered. It's up to you whether you go and rewrite the chart; I wouldn't, but I wouldn't let loose a stream of invective either.

As with your medical colleagues, tell other members of the team when you think they are doing well. A simple, 'I thought you handled that difficult situation well', means a lot to you or any of your medical or other colleagues. It also makes them much more likely to be receptive should you want to suggest they might do anything better.

General practitioners

- Don't forget the general practitioner.
- Ask the general practitioner for their views.
- Remember that general practitioners also work under stress.
- Don't give the general practitioner a ridiculous viva.

Most patients have a general practitioner. Don't forget them. If a patient dies in hospital, call the patient's doctor without delay. A message on the answerphone is all that is required. It is unacceptable if the first that your colleague knows about this is when they are accosted by distressed relatives.

There is a saying in the wine business: 'one glance at the label is worth years in the trade'. In a case where things don't seem to add up, always give the patient's doctor a call.

Many hospital doctors forget that there are certainly more frail and ill people at home than there are in hospital. It is also generally true that those working in primary care are closer to the problems of their patients, and the tongues of the relatives, than are doctors based in hospital. General practitioners often work under stress, as do doctors in hospital; most do not rush to phone to request for emergency medical admission without reasonable cause. It is sensible to remember this.

Remember also that general practitioners may be working in conditions that are 'less than ideal'. It is difficult to perform a rectal examination in a small, dark, cold caravan when the patient is huddled in a corner wearing eight layers of clothes, clutching their belly and moaning. The patient clearly needs to be sent to hospital without delay, and to give the referring doctor a lecture on the requirements for a satisfactory medical examination and referral is naive, stupid and 'likely to lead to a break down of good communications between the community and hospital services'.

1 Teamwork in medicine website http://www.gmc-uk.org/n_hance/med_ed/teamwork.htm
2 Reason J. Human error: models and management. *BMJ* 2000; 320: 768–770.

4.2 The 'modern' health service

 Doctors and hospitals must be able to demonstrate good practice, not just assert it.

 If you're in a hole, stop digging and shout for help.

Most doctors have always tried to the best of their ability to practise good medicine. Of course they must continue do so, but this is no longer enough. Recent events concerning heart surgery in Bristol, Mr Ledward, and very much more substantially by the case of Dr Shipman, have concentrated the public's and the politicians' minds to demand more of the medical profession. There is a need, which will not go away, to demonstrate in an open fashion that:

- health care is of a high and uniform standard across the country
- each and every individual clinician is continuing to practise in a competent manner.

How is this to be done? There is no easy answer. A colossal amount has been written; new words have been created; a month never goes by without another set of guidelines being produced by someone or other; it is easy to get thoroughly confused. The processes are developing, rather than developed, and whatever is written now is almost certain to be out of date by the time it is read. Many questions remain unanswered:

- Outcome—most important: will these new processes really improve the care of patients? If they do, then they are justified on that basis alone.
- Time—if we are all to do things we don't do at the moment, who will do the work we're doing now when we're gone?
- Money—who will pay for anything that needs to be paid for? If it has to come out of money otherwise used for patient care, can we really believe that it will be better spent on something else?
- Failure—what, precisely, will be the response if a problem with a particular hospital or an individual doctor is identified?

National standards

With the stated intention of providing a high and uniform standard of health care across the country, and ensuring that money is not wasted on ineffective treatments, the government has recently introduced, or stimulated others to introduce, a number of new initiatives.

National Service Frameworks (NSF)

These set national standards and define service models for a specific service or care group: that for coronary heart disease was the first to be published in March 2000; those for older people and for diabetes are the next in line. The intention is that one new National Service Framework will be developed each year.

If the National Service Framework for coronary heart disease [1] is representative of the style of these documents, they will be very specific in their demands.

 Hospitals ... should undertake an annual clinical audit that allows them to estimate the items listed ... below ...
Number and percentage of patients discharged from hospital with a diagnosis of acute myocardial infarction:
(a) prescribed aspirin
(b) prescribed β-blocker
(c) prescribed ACE inhibitor
(d) prescribed statin.
(National Service Frameworks [1])

Clinical Effectiveness and Evaluation Unit (CEEU)

The Royal College of Physicians has created a Clinical Effectiveness and Evaluation Unit [2]. Its first three online reports are on:

- Acute myocardial infarction core data set (prepared on behalf of the National Service Framework for coronary heart disease)
- Lung cancer core data set
- National clinical guidelines for stroke.

National Institute of Clinical Excellence (NICE)

This has the role of examining contentious (and expensive) treatments and advising on whether or not they should be provided under the NHS and, if so, to whom [3]. The first five appraisals completed deal with:

- Zanamivir (Relenza)
- Removal of wisdom teeth
- Prostheses for primary hip replacement
- Use of taxanes for ovarian cancer
- Guidance on coronary artery stents in the treatment of ischaemic heart disease.

Commission for Health Improvement (CHI)

This has the duty of inspecting and monitoring quality in NHS hospitals and primary care services [4]. Amongst its aims are:

- To provide national leadership to develop and disseminate clinical governance principles

• To conduct a rolling programme of reviews of clinical governance arrangements, visiting Trusts/Health Authorities every 4 years.

Clinical governance

Clinical governance means demonstrating in an open fashion that individual medical practitioners are continuing in competent clinical practice [5–7].

Key components have been set out in the document 'Physicians maintaining good medical practice: clinical governance and self-regulation' (Royal College of Physicians, London). The issues addressed are likely to become increasingly important for doctors everywhere and although the particular solutions found may differ from place to place, the fundamentals are not likely to vary greatly.

Appraising

What is the doctor supposed to do, and how are they doing? What is the doctor's job plan? What is going well? What are the obstacles and concerns? Appraisal is not supposed to be confrontational and is separate from disciplinary processes. It is standard practice in many other professions/businesses and hence fashionable. Most live to tell the tale, but external evidence of effectiveness of the process ('because of the introduction of an appraisal system, a certain hospital worked much better') is not available.

Developing

How can the doctor prove that they're keeping up to date?
• Continuing medical education (CME)/continuing professional development.
• Regularly updated personal development plan.

Reviewing

How can the doctor and the service they work for show that they treat their patients as well as they should do (and aren't worse than everybody else)?
• Participation in national audit.
• Peer-led service review.

There can be few objections in principle: the practice largely remains to be seen. However, it should be admitted that the power of the devices listed above is limited. For example, a reasonable person looking from the outside might judge a doctor as likely to be competent as follows: 'they've got lots of CME points, they must be concerned with keeping up to date; they must be a good doctor'. They might, in fact, be a complete lunatic.

Each doctor should know their limitations and ask for advice appropriately. This can be summarized: if you're in a hole, stop digging and shout for help.

Revalidation

In November 1998 the General Medical Council backed a proposal that all doctors on their register must be able to demonstrate—on a regular basis—that they are keeping themselves up to date and remain fit to practise in their chosen field. This is revalidation [8,9].

Poor performance

If you are aware that you have a problem of any sort that significantly impairs your ability to work as a doctor, you are obliged to discuss this with the Trust's Medical Director (or you may prefer first to discuss it with the College's Standards Adviser).

If you are aware that a colleague is performing poorly, then you should notify the Trust's Medical Director (or you may prefer first to discuss it with the College's Standards Adviser). This is not a matter of 'tale telling'; to quote the rubric, 'failure to do so could lead to disciplinary action'.

Whilst the details are again parochial, the important points are general. Patients can be harmed by doctors who perform poorly. The medical profession should not 'cover up' in such cases. The public needs protection and any doctors concerned must be offered appropriate help to improve their practice [5,10].

1 National Service Frameworks. Available at http://www.doh.gov.uk/nsf
2 Clinical Effectiveness and Evaluation Unit. Available at http://www.rcplondon.ac.uk/pubs/ceeu_online_home.htm
3 National Institute of Clinical Excellence. Available at http://www.nice.org.uk/appraisals
4 Commission for Health Improvement. Available at http://www.doh.gov.uk/chi/index.htm
5 Physicians maintaining good medical practice: Clinical governance and self-regulation. RCP, February 1999.
6 *Clinical Governance: Quality in the New NHS*. NHSE, March 1999.
7 Miles A, Hampton J, Hurwitz B, eds. *NICE, CHI and the NHS Reforms: Enabling Excellence or Imposing Control?* London: Key Advances Ltd, 2000. Centre for Health Services Research, Department of Health Sciences, University of East London, London E15 4LZ.
8 The details of how revalidation will work are not yet finalized: the Council of the GMC established a Revalidation Steering Group (RSG) to develop the project. Details of progress can be found at http://www.gmc-uk.org/n_hance/good/reval.htm
9 Smith R. The GMC: where now? *BMJ* 2000; 320: 1356.
10 *Supporting Doctors, Protecting Patients.* A consultation paper on preventing, recognizing and dealing with poor performance of doctors in the NHS in England. Department of Health, PO Box 777, London SE1 6XH. Available at http://www.doh.gov.uk/cmoconsult1.htm

4.3 Rationing beds

- It is a managerial and not a medical decision to close the hospital.
- If you think things are becoming unsafe, let the appropriate manager and senior doctor know.

Despite many pontifications and much posturing in high places, all doctors working in hospitals know that they don't have enough beds, and spend lots of time trying to force quarts into pint pots. The brunt is always borne in the places where emergencies come into hospitals: the A&E departments, and the medical admissions units. Most have a policy (fantasy) that says something like: 'when the patient has been assessed and a decision made to admit, they will be transferred to the most appropriate bed'.

The fact of the matter is that there usually isn't an appropriate bed. The case of gastrointestinal bleeding can't go to a ward specializing in gastroenterology, or to the ward of the team on take. Indeed, there often isn't a bed at all 'at the moment', and the patient has to remain in the admissions unit. This becomes overcrowded, patients land up on trolleys in the corridors and in wheelchairs when the trolleys run out. Everyone becomes short of oxygen, tempers get frayed and then another GP rings up.

How can this be managed? On the day clinical priorities must be established, those who are sickest need to be dealt with first, along with those who need particular treatments without delay, e.g. thrombolysis in myocardial infarction. In the longer term, there are discussions to be had with colleagues, management and politicians about the running of emergency medical services—but here we drift away from the immediate problem of 'how do you cope?' When the unit is full to busting, how do you handle the call from the next GP?

The ground rules should be:
- It is a managerial decision to close a hospital to admissions, not a medical one.
- Make sure that the appropriate consultant and manager know if you think that the place is becoming, or going to become, so crowded as to be unsafe.
- Enter into reasonable discussions with the GPs and offer alternatives to admission (next day clinics, speak to specialist registrar, etc.) if these are available and appropriate.
- If a GP rings about someone who clearly needs to be in hospital, don't try to fob them off. If your hospital is open—say 'send them'. If your hospital is closed—say 'we're closed'. Don't say 'it's very busy' and whine.
- Don't get angry. Don't take it personally. Do your best, and then go home.

Not having enough beds is one of the main mechanisms of rationing health care: it is a brilliantly effective and simple method of stopping doctors and nurses from treating patients and spending money. There are many other variations on the rationing theme, but here is not the place for lengthy discussion of the subtleties.

4.4 Stress

- Everyone has to find his or her own method of coping with stress.
- Make sure the method chosen doesn't upset others.

Most jobs can be stressful at some time or another, and this certainly applies to the business of being a doctor. This isn't the place for a treatise on 'How Doctors Should Cope With Stress', but everyone has to find a method of coping that works for them. It is important that the method chosen doesn't upset other people.

If you find yourself beginning to behave in a manner which makes a headless chicken look organized, or feel as though you're about to scream, then you should consider doing the following:
- Take yourself off for 3 minutes: there are very few situations when you cannot do this—cardiac arrest or severe circulatory collapse, acute upper airway obstruction, tension pneumothorax, (consultant ward round).
- Take a few deep breaths.
- Think about the things you have to do.
- Think about whether you can or should ask anyone else to help you.
- Go back and tackle the most important thing first.

When you leave the hospital at the end of the shift, think for 2 minutes about why you got in a pickle and plan how you will reduce the chances of this happening next time. The solution may be an 'internal' one, but you may need to speak to other people.

Being a doctor is a challenging task and all the more interesting for that. Different doctors do very different jobs: the child psychiatrist and the cardiothoracic surgeon rarely speak to each other and may well belong to different species (I know of no case where the two have produced fertile offspring). All doctors, however, have some aspects of their work in common and a range of these have been discussed in this section of the *Medical Masterclass*. The issues are universal, although the particular solutions suggested may not suit everyone. However, if you have read this far, you will at least have given some consideration to the matters discussed and will hopefully have thought of better answers for yourself.

Pain Relief and Palliative Care

AUTHOR:
G.N. Rudd

SECTION EDITOR AND EDITOR-IN-CHIEF:
J.D. Firth

1 Clinical presentations

1.1 Back pain

Case study

A 37-year-old woman who finished radical treatment for stage II carcinoma of the cervix 6 months ago attends your clinic. She is married with a 3-year-old son and her treatment included Weitheim's hysterectomy, external beam radiation and intracavity caesium. She has experienced increasing severe low-back pain over the last month, which has not been helped by coproxamol.

Clinical approach

Your main concern is to decide whether the pain is associated with her carcinoma of the cervix. The other common possibility in this age group is musculoskeletal pain due to a mechanical cause. It is also important to consider referred pain from another site.

 Do not assume that the pain must be associated with the carcinoma. The common differential diagnoses of low-back pain in a young patient are shown below.

Mechanical
Causes are:
- non-specific unknown aetiology
- prolapsed intravertebral disc
- spinal abnormalities—spinal stenosis or spondylosis.

Inflammatory
Causes are:
- infections
- ankylosing spondylitis
- sacroilitis
- arachnoiditis.

Other causes
These include:
- bone metastases (clearly much more likely than usual in this case)
- myeloma
- intrathecal tumours
- referred pain, e.g. peptic ulcer
- metabolic causes, e.g. osteomalacia.

History of the presenting problem

An accurate history of the pain may give important clues to the aetiology. Ask:
- Where is it?
- Is it in more than one site?
- What is it like? (ask the patient to use descriptive terms, e.g. 'burning')
- How severe is it? (a score out of 10 can be helpful)
- Is it getting worse?
- Is it constant?
- What precipitates it?
- Can she sleep at night?

Malignant pain may be in multiple sites. It is often progressive and constant, although some pains may disappear strangely at times. Pain is often severe at night, although some patients may find comfortable positions in which to sleep.

Does the pain radiate? Pain that radiates down the leg and particularly below the knee is usually caused by nerve root compression. Patients may describe stabbing or burning pain radiating down the leg.

How is she otherwise? Are there any other symptoms? Ask specifically ask about weight, appetite and sweating. Loss of weight, poor appetite and sweating would all suggest a malignant cause.

Treatment of the pain

Ask the patient:
- What have you tried to relieve the pain?
- Ask specifically about medically prescribed drugs, physical treatments and homeopathic remedies.
- Has anything helped?

It is not possible to give good advice without knowing exactly what has been used in the past, and whether it has worked.

Relevant past medical history

Ask the patient:
- Have you had anything like this before?
- Have you had any other previous illness?

A patient with malignant disease may have other reasons for symptoms and it is important to pursue alternative possibilities for pain in this case.

Social history

Ask the following:
• How has she been coping physically at home with her 3-year-old son?
• Enquire what impact her initial diagnosis had on her and her family and how her husband has coped.
• Ask if she was able to resume sexual relations after her initial treatment.
• Is there any other social support?
• How will they cope financially if she is in hospital and her husband needs to take time off to look after their child?

All these are things that the patient may be worried about, but not feel comfortable about introducing into conversation with the doctor, feeling that 'the doctor wouldn't be interested in these problems'. It is true that doctors may not have the time or the expertise to tackle these issue themselves, but it is important that these enquiries are made, because useful help and support can be given by allied professionals (counsellors, social workers, etc.).

Examination

General impressions are very important:
• observe if the patient is sitting comfortably
• is she relaxed and smiling, or does she look as though she is in pain?
• does she look ill?
• has she lost weight?

Musculoskeletal and neurological assessment

Since the presentation is with back pain, concentrate initially on musculoskeletal and neurological assessment. Are there areas of tenderness?
• Start gently; ask the patient to pinpoint them.
• Is the lower lumbar spine tender?
Examine the peripheral nervous system, looking for:
• signs of lumbar or sacral nerve root compression; and
• areas of hyperalgesia as well as reduced sensation.
Specifically:
• loss of sensation in the inner calf
• weakness of inversion of the foot
• loss of knee reflex.
Signs of nerve root compression would almost certainly indicate malignant involvement of the spine or paraspinal tissues in this case.

General examination

Because the main concern is the possibility of recurrent malignancy, some features of the general examination are particularly important. Look carefully for:

• Lymphadenopathy
• Anaemia
• Abdominal/pelvic masses
• Lung pathology.
The presence of any of these features would strongly suggest recurrent or disseminated malignancy.

Approach to investigations and management

Investigations

To look for evidence to support the diagnosis of disseminated malignancy (e.g. bone metastases) or complications of recurrent pelvic disease (e.g. urinary obstruction leading to renal failure) initiate the following:
• Blood count
• ESR or CRP
• Urea, electrolytes, liver function tests
• Alkaline phosphatase—may be elevated with bone secondaries
• Bone scan—may be helpful to exclude widespread bone secondaries.
To look for evidence of local tumour recurrence take:
• Plain radiograph of the lumbar spine and pelvis—ask for lateral and anteroposterior views as the first abnormality seen with bone secondaries is loss of the pedicles
• MRI scan—will show soft-tissue mass as well as bone disease and is often a very useful investigation.

In this case, MRI confirmed the clinical suspicion of local tumour recurrence (Fig. 1).

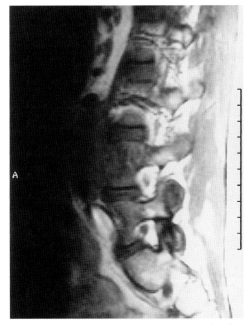

Fig. 1 MRI scan showing a soft-tissue mass at the L3/L4 level with involvement of the vertebral body of L4.

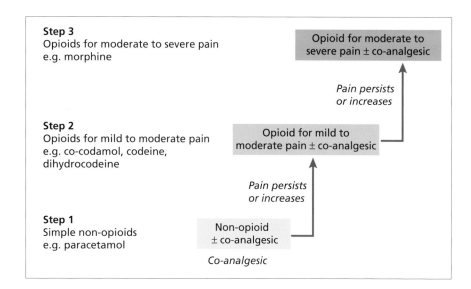

Fig. 2 WHO analgesic ladder.

Management

Pain was treated as per the World Health Organization (WHO) analgesic ladder (Fig. 2). Dihydrocodeine did not relieve it and she was therefore started on short-acting morphine with a non-steroidal anti-inflammatory drug (NSAID) and her dose requirements titrated. This improved her back pain but she continued to experience pain in her leg. Amitriptyline was added with some effect. However, the anticholinergic side effects were severe and she was changed to carbamazepine. She was stabilized on long-acting morphine and carbamazepine, but was unable to have further radiotherapy because of previous treatment.

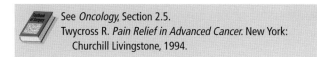

See *Oncology*, Section 2.5.
Twycross R. *Pain Relief in Advanced Cancer.* New York: Churchill Livingstone, 1994.

1.2 Nausea and vomiting

Case study

A 45-year-old teacher is referred to your unit. She had presented to her GP with vague abdominal symptoms 18 months previously. Six months later, she was found to have stage III carcinoma of the ovary. She was treated with total abdominal hysterectomy and bilateral salpingo-oophorectomy and chemotherapy. However, she relapsed rapidly after the end of first-line chemotherapy and had a minimal response to second-line chemotherapy. She is now vomiting four to six times a day.

Clinical approach

Is the vomiting due to the cancer or due to something else?

Is vomiting due to ovarian cancer?
• Bowel obstruction.
• Obstructive nephropathy with renal failure.
• Hypercalcaemia.

Is vomiting due to something else?
• Intercurrent gastrointestinal infection.
• Drug effect.
• Constipation.

History of the presenting problem

Details of the vomiting are necessary:
• Can she keep anything down? Is she thirsty? If she can keep nothing down and feels thirsty, she is likely to be very dehydrated.
• Does she regurgitate rather than vomit? If she brings back unaltered food, then she is likely to have oesophageal obstruction.
• Does she have a feeling of fullness and then vomit copious amounts? This would suggest gastric outlet obstruction.
• When did she last open her bowels? Does she have associated abdominal pain? Severe constipation, often induced by opiate analgesics, is a common cause of vomiting. Absolute constipation and severe colicky abdominal pain, temporarily relieved by vomiting, would be typical of intestinal obstruction.
• Has she started any new drugs, e.g. metronidazole/first few days of opiates/selective serotonin reuptake inhibitors (SSRIs)? Any of these could cause nausea and vomiting.
• Is there anyone else close to her with similar symptoms? Patients with cancer are not protected from infective gastroenteritis.

Other relevant history

Check whether this has happened before, and if so, why?

Examination

The important aspects are described below.

Is she frail?

Although not easy to define, it is important to recognize frailty and it is not difficult to do so. Those who are frail are likely to die sooner rather than later. The doctor needs to appreciate this, and to behave accordingly in discussion of prognosis and treatment options with the patient and their relatives or carers.

Is she dehydrated?

Postural hypotension and a low jugular venous pulse indicate intravascular volume depletion. Reduced tissue turgor and dry lips and tongue suggest dehydration (reduction in total body water).

What does her oral cavity look like?

If the lips, tongue and mouth are parched and cracked, this can cause terrible discomfort and prevent the patient from eating or drinking adequately even if there is no other impediment to this. Careful nursing attention to the mouth can provide great relief. White plaques suggest candida.

What can you find abdominally?

Is she obstructed? Has she got ascites? Look for a distended, tender abdomen with high-pitched bowel sounds to diagnose obstruction; and shifting dullness to diagnose ascites.

Approach to investigations and management

Investigations

A detailed history and examination should indicate the aetiology and, if there is bowel obstruction, whether it is 'high gastric outflow' or lower bowel obstruction.

An abdominal radiograph may be helpful in determining whether or not there is obstruction, and the level of that obstruction.

Urea and electrolytes—to determine the degree of dehydration (urea rises disproportionately to creatinine: why? see *Physiology*, Section 6), and look for hypokalaemia (why does vomiting cause hypokalaemia? see *Physiology*, Section 6) and renal failure.

Liver function tests—may be abnormal if there are liver metastases.

Calcium—may be elevated in malignancies with or without bone metastases.

Management

 Your management may depend on her functional state:
- Can she transfer or walk?
- Ask how she spends her day.
- Is she enjoying any aspect of her life?

 Discuss management options with the patient:
- Would she consider a surgical option?
- How does she react to the possibility of an ileostomy?

Intravascular volume depletion should be corrected with intravenous 0.9% saline (with potassium supplementation if needed); dehydration with alternating 0.9% saline and 5% dextrose, or using 0.45% saline and 2.5% dextrose.

The patient was rehydrated and given stool softeners. Pain was treated with antispasmodics (hyoscine butylbromide). High-dose intravenous dexamethasone was started. Five days later, she opened her bowels and her vomiting started to settle. She was maintained on low-dose dexamethasone and a combined stimulant/softener laxative.

She re-presented 6 weeks later with worsening symptoms and a request for surgical intervention. An ileostomy was carried out with improvement of symptoms.

 See *Oncology*, Section 2.5.

1.3 Breathlessness

Case study

A 70-year-old woman is admitted from A&E. Fifteen years previously, carcinoma of the breast was treated by lumpectomy, radiotherapy and tamoxifen. She now has lung metastases which have progressed despite progesterones, aromatase inhibitors and epirubin. Her breathlessness has now worsened.

Clinical approach

Your main concern is to identify reversible causes of increased breathlessness. If there is no reversible cause, you need to try and palliate her symptoms as much as possible.

Any cause of breathlessness can affect a patient with cancer, but those that are particularly common include:
- anaemia
- anxiety
- ascites
- bronchial obstruction
- chest infection
- lymphangitis
- pleural effusion
- pneumothorax
- pulmonary embolism
- pericardial effusion
- superior vena caval obstruction.

History of the presenting problem

How bad is the breathlessness? Does it limit her walking and if so, how far can she walk?

A detailed history is necessary to establish the cause:

- When is she breathless? Does it fluctuate? Does she wheeze? Asthma and anxiety are common causes of fluctuating breathlessness. Wheezing may be due to bronchial obstruction, asthma or cardiac failure.
- Has it worsened suddenly or gradually? Breathlessness that comes on suddenly (in an instant) is more likely to be due to pneumothorax or bronchial obstruction, sometimes pulmonary embolism. Most of the causes listed above are likely to cause symptoms that worsen over days or weeks.
- Does she expectorate sputum? Suggests infection.
- Does she have haemoptysis? If haemoptysis is massive, this suggests erosion of bronchi by secondaries. Also consider pulmonary embolism.
- Is there any chest pain? Pleuritic pain may be due to pulmonary embolism or pneumonia. Metastatic invasion of pleura and/or pleural effusion are more likely to cause a dull, heavy pain.
- Does she have any ankle swelling? This is often found with cardiac failure, caval obstruction, venous thromboembolism, ascites or hypoproteinaemia.

Other relevant history

Are there any coexisting problems which are contributing to the dyspnoea? It is important to ask about general health and social circumstances.

- How does she feel when she is at rest?
- Are there any other problems?
- Is she eating?
- How does she usually spend her day?
- Does she have relatives and friends?

All these are relevant when it comes to deciding how best to treat.

Examination

 General impressions are important and will determine management.
- Is she cyanosed?
- How distressing is her dyspnoea?
- Is she frail and cachectic?

General examination

Look for other features of disseminated or locally invasive malignancy:
- Anaemia
- Lymphadenopathy
- Signs of superior vena caval obstruction—swelling of face, neck and arms; plethoric cyanotic facies; non-pulsatile engorement of veins; collateral vessels over the surface of the shoulders, scapulae and upper chest; brush venules over the chest wall.

Check the oral cavity (see Section 1.2, p. 28).

Respiratory assessment

Particularly look for:
- Collapse/consolidation
- Pleural effusion
- Pleural rub
- Wheeze.

Cardiovascular assessment

Consider:
- Is her breathlessness due to heart failure?
- Does she have a pericardial effusion? (Look for: absent apex beat, faint heart sounds, pericardial rub, and in tamponade, raised venous pressure, hypotension, pulsus paradoxus: see *Cardiology*, Section 1.8.)

In this case, examination revealed a patient who looked well at rest, but became breathless on transferring from bed to chair; the following were also revealed:
- A moderate left-sided pleural effusion
- A moderate inspiratory left-sided wheeze.

Approach to investigations and management

Investigations

 Avoid unnecessary investigations, but do investigate appropriately:
- Check blood count to confirm clinical impression.
- Chest radiograph to confirm pleural effusion and assess if there is progression of pulmonary metastases.

Management

Discussion with patient and family, explaining that the disease had progressed and emphasis would be on symptomatic measures. Two litres of pleural fluid was aspirated with some improvement in dyspnoea. Exercise tolerance improved with bronchodilators and nebulizers were started. Oxygen was used when needed and was arranged by the GP at home. Relaxation and breathing techniques were taught to counteract intermittent mild dyspnoeic/panic attacks at rest. The patient was referred to an occupational therapist to maximize the limited period of independent existence at home.

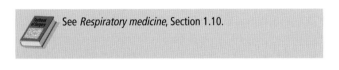

See *Respiratory medicine*, Section 1.10.

1.4 Confusion

Case study

A 78-year-old man is admitted from A&E as an emergency —dehydrated and confused. He had been found wandering by neighbours, who called an ambulance.

Clinical approach

Your main concern is to ascertain the cause of his confusion and try and piece together his previous medical history. It would be helpful to know whether his confusion is of recent onset. He clearly cannot tell you this: you need to obtain the history from someone else (partner, relatives, carers, friends) if at all possible. His hospital notes are not immediately available so you proceed to examine him.

Examination

General impressions are important:
- He is frail, cachectic and distressed
- He seems to be in discomfort in the bed
- He is dehydrated.
  Also:
- There is oral candida and angular stomatitis
- He has a hard lymph node in the right supraclavicular fossa
- He has a laparotomy scar and a tender mass in the right upper quadrant compatible with hepatomegaly
- Cardiovascular and respiratory systems are normal
- There is no obvious focal neurology.

The obvious clinical suspicion is that he has disseminated malignancy.

Common causes of confusion in patients with cancer are listed in Table 1.

Table 1 Common causes of confusion in the patient with cancer.

Infective	Urinary tract
	Chest
	Fungal
Metabolic	Hypercalcaemia
	Hyponatraemia
	Liver failure
	Uraemia
	Hypoxia from any cause
Drug induced	Opioids (overdose or withdrawal)
	Sedatives, e.g. benzodiazepines
	Cimetidine, carbamazepine
	Corticosteroids
	Alcohol withdrawal
	Hyoscine
Neurological	Dementia
	Brain metastases (rarely)
	Post-ictal
Psychiatric	Paranoid delusional state
Other	Urinary retention
	Constipation

Approach to investigations and management

Investigations

You investigate him for the common reversible causes of confusion.
- Blood count—he is mildly anaemic
- Urea and electrolytes—the urea is elevated at 13.6 mmol/L
- Liver and bone blood tests—he is hypercalcaemic, with his calcium at 3.2 mmol/L (what are the causes of hypercalcaemia?—see *Endocrinology*, Section 1.2)
- Dipstick test of urine
- Blood and urine cultures are sent
- Pulse oximetry—his saturation on air is 97%
- Chest radiograph—this is a poor quality film, but shows no diagnostic features.

Management

The team, after consultation with relatives, decides that the hypercalcaemia should be treated and he is therefore given 0.9% saline and disodium pamidronate. Oral candida is treated with fluconazole.

The hospital notes are obtained, showing that 3 years previously he had a hemicolectomy for cancer of the colon. There is no mention of confusion at his last visit to the surgical clinic, but it was noted that his condition was generally poor. You are uncertain whether to investigate the patient further and he remains agitated and distressed.

His confusion improves after 3 days but he remains bed bound and weak. A request is made for an ultrasound examination of the liver with the intention of confirming the clinical suspicion of disseminated malignancy, but before this is done he worsens and becomes acutely agitated again.

Another investigation that might be considered in this situation is a CT scan of the brain, but cerebral metastases are unlikely in the absence of any focal neurological signs and it is unlikely that the patient could co-operate adequately to undergo scanning without sedation/anaesthesia.

- Does he have recurrent hypercalcaemic symptoms?
- Does he have an infection?
- Is he in pain and unable to express this?
- Is this agitation associated with his dying?

Further management

After discussion with all members of the medical and nursing team involved in his care, the decision is made that the diagnosis of disseminated malignancy and terminal illness is clear, despite the absence of histological confirmation, and that further investigation or aggressive attempts to prolong life would not be kind or sensible.

From your previous discussions with his relatives you know that they are aware of the situation and would not want his distress to be prolonged. You explain your view of the situation to them, can see that they approve of the line you are taking, and say that the medical decision is not to pursue further investigation, to relieve distress with medication as needed, and to ensure that he passes away as peacefully as possible.

His agitation is managed successfully with subcutaneous midazolam. He dies the next day.

See *Endocrinology*, Section 1.2.
See *General clinical issues*, Section 3.
Twycross R. *Pain Relief in Advanced Cancer.* New York: Churchill Livingstone, 1994.
Twycross R. *Symptom Management in Advanced Cancer,* 2nd edn. Oxford: Radcliffe Medical Press, 1997.

2 Diseases and treatments

2.1 Pain

Aetiology

Pain is an unpleasant sensory and emotional experience associated with actual or potential tissue damage, or described in terms of such damage (International Association for Study of Pain 1986).

The classification of pain is contentious. Twycross classifies pain as 'nociceptive or neuropathic with subdivisions of both into either physiological (functional) and pathological and then further into somatic vs visceral'. Useful terminology for pain is shown in Table 2.

Pain in cancer patients may be due to:
- cancer, either primary or secondary
- debility, e.g. bed sores, stiffness from inactivity
- treatment, e.g. vincristine neuropathy, thoracotomy scar pain
- concurrent disorder, e.g. arthritis, osteoporosis.

A simplified schema of the neuroanatomy and neurophysiology of pain and sites of action of some analgesics is shown in Fig. 3. There are nerve endings (nociceptors) in all tissues which when stimulated by noxious stimuli (mechanical, chemical or thermal) will give rise to pain.
- Different types of nerve fibres exist: A, B and C with α, β, δ and γ subcategories.
- A α, A γ and B are motor fibres; A β, A δ and C are sensory fibres.

Different nociceptors will give rise to different pains; for instance, the A δ will give rise to the first sharp pain of injury, while the C nociceptors will then produce a slow throbbing pain. The different types of pain are outlined in Table 3.

Epidemiology

Approximately 75% of patients with cancer experience pain at some time during their last year of life. Many patients have more than one type of pain.

Clinical presentation

Patients will present in many different ways. The concept of total pain acknowledges the distress a patient with a serious illness experiences and the contribution of psychological, social, spiritual and financial problems to their predicament.

Dying patients face multiple losses and anxieties, pain being one facet of their disease and often a constant reminder of their situation.

Case history example

A 43-year-old with advanced colorectal cancer experienced constant right upper quadrant liver capsular pain. He also admitted to financial and family worries. He had particular difficulty in telling his 11-year-old daughter that he was going to die. After he had been able to do this, he started to sleep at night and although never perfect, his pain control improved markedly.

Assessment of pain

A clear history and assessment of pain is the basis of treatment. Successful treatment therefore relies on knowledge of the aetiology and recognition that several types and sites of pain may coexist.

Pain history should include the following questions:
- When did it start?
- Where is it and does it radiate anywhere?
- What is the character of the pain?
- Is it constant or does it fluctuate?
- Does anything alleviate or exacerbate it?
- Which analgesics have been tried and what effect did they have?
- Are there any associated factors?

Table 2 Terminology of pain.

Terminology	Description
Nociception	The activity produced in the nervous system by potential or actual tissue-damaging stimuli
	Pain is the perception of nociception
Allodynia	Pain due to a stimulus that does not normally provoke pain
Hyperalgesia	Increased response to a stimulus that is normally painful
Hyperpathia	An increased reaction to a stimulus as well as an increased threshold

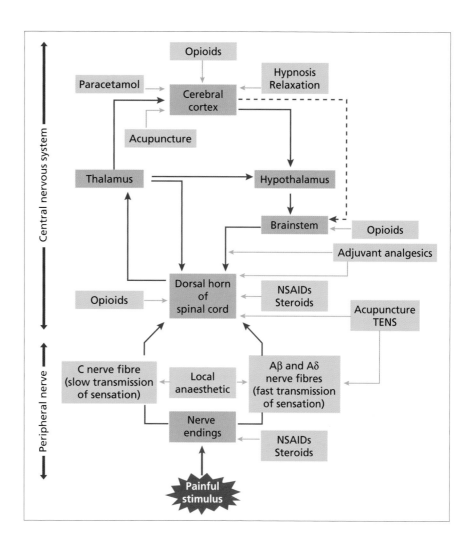

Fig. 3 A schema of the neuroanatomy of pain and the sites of action of different analgesic modalities. NSAIDs, non-steroidal anti-inflammatory drugs; TENS, transelectrical nerve stimulation.

- What effect does it have on your life?
- Do you have any particular fears or anxieties?

 More than anything else you should listen to the patient and believe them.

Table 3 Types of pain.

Type	Description
Somatic	This arises from damage to skin and deep tissues. It is usually localized and is often of an aching quality
Visceral	Arises from abdominal or thoracic viscera. Pain is often described as deep or pressure pain and is poorly localized
Neuropathic	This is due to nerve damage either in the peripheral or central nervous system. This may be described as 'burning' or 'stabbing' in quality. It often occurs in an area of abnormal or decreased sensation. Neuropathic pain may respond to opioids, but in many cases co-analgesic drugs are required

Physical signs

Assess the state of the patient's disease and note palpable evidence of disease spread. Palpate areas of pain to elicit tenderness, e.g. from bone secondaries. Examine the nervous system looking for signs of reduced power and abnormal sensation. Assess the reflexes.

 Remember that some pains are 'referred pain'.

Treatment

Rules for analgesic prescribing are shown in Fig. 2 (p. 27) and Table 4.
- Move up the ladder if the current step is ineffective.
- Give all medication regularly and by mouth unless unable to take oral medication.

Table 4 Rules for analgesic prescribing.

- Continuous pain requires regular analgesics to prevent re-occurrence
- Start simply and follow analgesic ladder
- Consider co-analgesics
- Be patient and give each drug a therapeutic trial at the appropriate dose
- Anticipate and treat side effects
- Give drugs by mouth unless patients are unable to tolerate this route, i.e. vomiting, dysphagia

• It may be appropriate to add a co-analgesic before moving up the analgesic ladder.

Opioids

Morphine

Morphine is an extremely useful drug that should be titrated for each individual patient. There is no upper limit on dose prescribed.

TITRATION OF MORPHINE

The initial dose depends on previous analgesia, age and coexisting medical problems, particularly renal failure, in which opiates and their metabolites accumulate.

Most patients should be started on 5–10 mg orally 4-hourly, with the same dose prescribed as a 'breakthrough' or 'rescue dose' whenever needed. Once drug requirements are constant, the patient can be converted to long-acting morphine (MST, MXL) or fentanyl patches. It is imperative that short-acting morphine preparations continue to be prescribed for breakthrough pain and increased in step with the long-acting morphine preparation. They should be given at one-sixth of the long-acting dose.

Case history example

The palliative care team was asked to review urgently a young patient with severe pain. She had been admitted the previous night with worsening dyspnoea and pain due to metastatic carcinoma of the breast with bone (Fig. 4) and lung secondaries. She had previously been stable on fentanyl 400 µg/h. The covering SHO continued the fentanyl patch, but recognizing her difficulty with oral medication charted diamorphine 2.5–5 mg s.c. prn for her breakthrough medication. The correct dose was 40 mg s.c. prn—see below.

Long-acting opioids in frequent use

MORPHINE SULPHATE CONTINUS

Twelve-hourly preparation in tablets or granules which can be made into a suspension.

MXL

Once-daily preparation of long-acting morphine in capsules.

FENTANYL

Synthetic opioid as a transdermal patch used every 3 days. Variable pharmacokinetics: some patients may need to

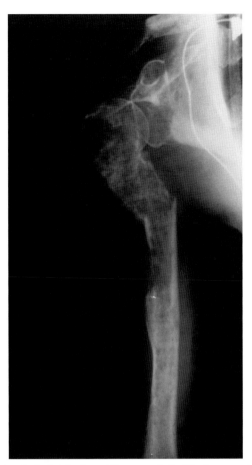

Fig. 4 A pathological fracture of the upper shaft of the humerus due to multiple lytic deposits.

change patches every 2 days. Useful for patients with difficult constipation or who are unable to take tablets. A patch supplying 25 µg fentanyl per hour provides equivalent analgesia to 90 mg oral morphine sulphate over 24 hours.

HYDROMORPHONE

Hydromorphone has only recently been available in the UK and is thought to have fewer side effects than morphine. 1.3 mg of hydromorphone is equivalent to 10 mg of morphine sulphate.

OXYCODONE

Available for many years as a suppository; long- and short-acting preparations are now available. 5 mg of oxycodone is equivalent to 10 mg of morphine sulphate.

METHADONE

Useful for patients for neuropathic pain. Accumulates, therefore should be used with specialist supervision. The potency compared to morphine increases with multiple doses and is approximately 5–10 times as potent as oral morphine.

DEXTROMORAMIDE

A potent drug but use is limited by its short action of 2 hours. Excellent for short and painful procedures, e.g. dressing changes. 1 mg of dextromoramide is equivalent to 3 mg of morphine sulphate, however duration of action is shorter.

DIAMORPHINE

The opioid of choice for parenteral use due to great solubility. It can be given intravenously, intramuscularly or subcutaneously. It should be used when a patient is unable to absorb oral medication. It is two to three times more potent than morphine.

Case history example

A 65-year-old man with renal cell carcinoma and bone metastases was admitted because of general deterioration in his condition. He was pain-free but had increasing difficulty in swallowing medication, which included MST 90 mg p.o. twice daily. He was converted to a 24-hour diamorphine syringe driver with 60 mg diamorphine with 10 mg prn charted. He remained pain-free.

Side effects of opioids

The common side effects of opioids are shown in Table 5.

Fears about morphine and other opioids

Fears over the use of opioids are common in both patients and doctors. These concerns limit their appropriate prescription and unless discussed with the patient, may lead to non-compliance.

Patients are often fearful of morphine as they may think:
• 'then this must be the end'
• 'will I get addicted?'
• 'I will be drugged and unable to function properly'
• 'if I have morphine now, what will be left when I am really dying?'

Health care professionals are often concerned that they may:
• Induce respiratory depression
• Sedate the patient
• Cause confusion
• Cause addiction.

If used appropriately, none of these fears are justified, and the benefits of opioid prescription far outweigh the risks.

Co-analgesics for neuropathic pain

Neuropathic pain may be controlled with opiates; some will need the addition of co-analgesics.

Tricyclic antidepressants

These act by blocking the uptake of norepinephrine (noradrenaline) and serotonin. The analgesic effect is at a lower dose than used for depression and they exert their effect in approximately 4–5 days. Start at a low dose, e.g. amitriptyline 25 mg nocte, and gradually increase. Patients may experience transient drowsiness; some patients have intolerable anticholinergic side effects.

Anticonvulsants

Carbamazepine, sodium valproate, clonazepam, gabapentin (licensed in USA) are all used for neuropathic pain, particularly if shooting in nature. The mechanism of the analgesic effect is not fully understood. They should be started at low doses and gradually increased in order to minimize side effects. The analgesic effect of carbamazepine and sodium valproate develops in 3–5 days.

Corticosteroids

Corticosteroids can be useful in reducing inflammation around tumours, thereby relieving pressure on structures compressed, e.g. nerve roots, cerebral metastases. They may also have an effect on the prostaglandin pathway. Their usefulness is limited by side effects, but in the short term they can be a very effective co-analgesic.

Table 5 Common side effects of opioids.

Constipation	Occurs in almost all patients unless there is coexisting malabsorption. All patients should be treated prophylactically with stimulant laxative plus softener
Nausea	Affects one-third of patients, but in the majority is self-limiting within 1 week. Consider prophylactic antiemetics for 1 week
Drowsiness	Generally remits after a few days
Dry mouth	A common side effect
Hallucinations	Uncommon side effect, often visual and in peripheral field of vision
Nightmares	Vivid and unpleasant but uncommon
Myoclonic jerks	Occur particularly if overdosed, often confused with fits
Respiratory depression	Not a problem in patients in pain. However, occurs if pain is abolished, e.g. after a nerve block or radiotherapy

Other analgesics

NON-STEROIDAL ANTI-INFLAMMATORY DRUGS

The NSAIDs have analgesic and anti-inflammatory effects due to reduced prostaglandin synthesis. They are used frequently, particularly for bone pain. There are many different groups of NSAIDs and patients who fail to respond to a drug in one group may respond to another. New drugs which only inhibit one form of cyclo-oxygenase (COX-2 selective inhibitors) are now available, but there is no evidence of increased efficacy in patients with cancer.

OTHER AGENTS

Analgesics used by specialist teams include the following:
• Membrane-stabilizing drugs used for neuropathic pain, e.g. flecainide and mexilitine
• Ketamine—anaesthetic agent useful for neuropathic pain; the intravenous preparation is made into an oral solution
• Clonidine—used for neuropathic pain
• Bisphosphonates—for the treatment of bone metastases in patients with carcinoma of breast and myeloma. Their use for other cancers is being evaluated
• Antispasmodics—benzodiazepines/baclofen
• Cannabinoids—a group of drugs which has potential use for pain, nausea and breathlessness. Nabilone is the only synthetic cannabinoid available. Use is limited by side effects.

Other modalities of pain control

These include:
• Epidural and intrathecal opioids—for patients with severe side effects from opioids or pain requiring escalating doses of drugs
• Nerve blocks—for localized pain or pain from one nerve root. Initially injected with local anaesthetic ± steroids, if successful longer-term relief can be gained from neuroablation
• Palliative radiotherapy
• Chemotherapy
• TENS—electrical stimulation of A β fibres, which, according to the gate theory of pain, reduces the imprint from C fibres to the spinal cord
• Acupuncture
• Surgery—e.g. to stabilize a fracture of the spine or long bone, or prophylactically to prevent an impending fracture.

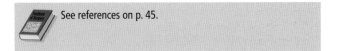
See references on p. 45.

2.2 Breathlessness

Aetiology

Breathlessness may be a direct symptom of a primary tumour or may occur because of lung secondaries (Fig. 5), lymphangitis carcinomatosis, pleural (Fig. 6) and pericardial effusions. The diaphragm may be splinted because of ascites or the lungs may be stiff because of mesothelioma.

There may be coexisting chronic lung disease, particularly in those with lung cancer, and many will have a degree of heart failure.

Acute infective events occur frequently in those who are ill, and there is a higher incidence of thrombosis and emboli in patients with cancer. Superior vena caval obstruction occurs in those with mediastinal disease.

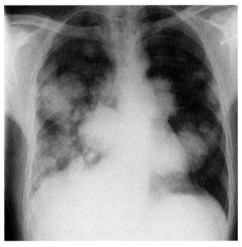

Fig. 5 Chest radiograph of a patient with diffuse pleuritic chest pain and breathlessness due to adenoid cystic carcinoma.

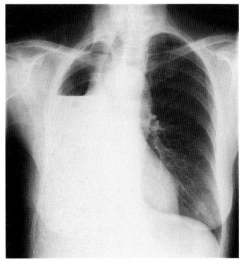

Fig. 6 Carcinoma of the bronchus with pleural effusion and traumatic pneumothorax.

Epidemiology

Breathlessness and cough are common symptoms in patients with cancer, with 47% reporting respiratory problems in their last year of life and 70% in the last 6 weeks.

Clinical presentation

Breathlessness is one of the most distressing symptoms that patients endure. It is frequently associated with panic as patients feel that they 'will never get another breath and are about to die'.

When I got home I sat in the chair and I lost all control of my breathing, I could not breathe at all. I just sat in a panic situation. I felt I was going to stop breathing at any moment … It was the most awful feeling I ever had and I have been through some awful situations in wartime, but I have never ever been as afraid as I was during this period.
(Patient with mesothelioma)

Patients may experience a gradual worsening of their breathing and exercise tolerance, or may present with intermittent wheeze and attacks of breathlessness.

When I did start running again, I found I was losing my capacity to breathe comfortably … After a while, I found I could only run up to 8 miles and I was absolutely shattered.
(75-year-old marathon runner with mesothelioma)

Insomnia is frequent and patients are often anxious. Breathlessness may be accompanied by cough and haemoptysis.

- Many patients are fearful of suffocating or drowning in their bronchial secretions. Asking about specific fears may be therapeutic in itself (see Section 2.9, p. 43).
- It may seem impossible to ask someone who is dying if they have any anxieties, but this can be done sensitively with something like—'I appreciate that you must have many fears and worries, but is there anything in particular that is preying on your mind?' (see Section 2.7, p. 42).

Physical signs

Look for:
- Anaemia
- Signs of right- or left-sided heart failure
- Bronchospasm, signs of collapse and consolidation
- Pleural effusions
- Pericardial effusions, pleural rubs
- Ascites.

Table 6 Treatment of breathlessness.

Treat reversible causes	Modify tumour, e.g. radiotherapy and chemotherapy/laser treatment Transfusion Anticoagulation Drainage of effusions or ascites Endobronchial or superior vena caval stents
Drug treatments	Bronchodilators Opioids Corticosteroids Benzodiazepines Antibiotics Diuretics
Other modalities	Oxygen Acupuncture Relaxation therapy Breathlessness clinics

Investigations

These should be purposeful, directed at reversible causes of breathlessness, or done to monitor or change specific tumour treatment.

Treatment

The treatment of breathlessness can be difficult. Success depends on determining the aetiology and treating any reversible causes, and then taking care to ameliorate physical symptoms and psychological distress as much as possible. Treatment modalities are shown in Table 6.

Stridor

Stridor is due to tracheal compression and requires emergency management. Give high-concentration oxygen and dexamethasone 16 mg i.v. Refer as an emergency to oncologists for radiotherapy if appropriate, or to head and neck surgeons for tracheostomy if indicated. Supportive treatment should include nebulized saline and sedation if appropriate.

See *Emergency medicine*, Sections 3.8 and 3.9.
See references on p. 45.

2.3 Nausea and vomiting

Aetiology

The emetic pathway is complex: many neuronal pathways are involved. A diagram of the pathways controlling

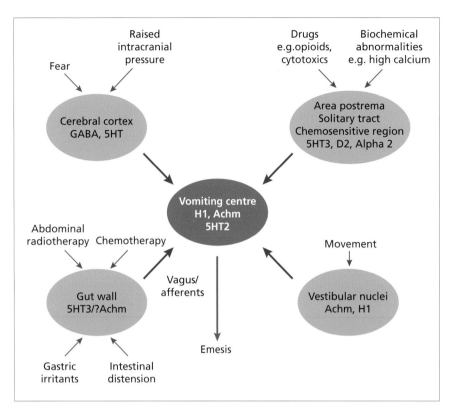

Fig. 7 Neural mechanisms controlling vomiting. Achm, muscarinic cholinergic; alpha 2, alpha adrenergic type 2; D2, dopamine type 2; GABA, gamma-aminobutyric acid; 5HT, 5-hydroxytryptamine; H1, histamine type 1.

Table 7 Causes of nausea and vomiting in patients with cancer.

Chemical	Drugs, e.g. digoxin, NSAIDs, opioids, ferrous sulphate, antiobiotics, chemotherapy
	Metabolic abnormalities, e.g. hypercalcaemia, uraemia, liver failure, ketoacidosis
	Toxins, e.g. food poisoning, ischaemic bowel
Gastric stasis	Drugs (anticholinergic effect), e.g. hyoscine, tricyclic antidepressants, opioids
	Autonomic failure, e.g. diabetes mellitus
	Gastric outflow compression by tumour or hepatomegaly
	Peptic ulceration/gastritis
Intestinal obstruction	Tumour
	Adhesions, e.g. postsurgical
	Fibrosis, e.g. postradiation
Irritation of visceral and gastrointestinal serosa	Constipation
	Liver secondaries
	Ureteric obstruction

vomiting is shown in Fig. 7. Common causes in cancer patients are listed in Table 7.

Epidemiology

Fifty-one per cent of patients with cancer will experience nausea and vomiting at some time in their last year of life, while 27% of those dying from another cause will suffer from it.

A careful history will elicit the aetiology, and understanding of the emetic pathway will allow the choice of appropriate antiemetic.

Treatment

Antiemetics in common use are listed in Table 8.

Twenty to 30% of patients may require two antiemetics. These should have different actions and should be compatible. In cases of unknown aetiology, low-dose methotrimeprazine (muscarinic cholinergic, dopamine type 2 and 5-hydroxytryptamine antagonist activity) can be useful.

Case history example

A 63-year-old man with carcinoma of the pancreas was producing large-volume vomits two or three times per day. He intermittently felt nauseated and was loathe to eat or drink. It was thought that he had gastric stasis due to partial outflow obstruction. He was started on metoclopramide with good effect. Six weeks later, his vomiting returned. Dexamethasone was added to the regime with improvement in his symptoms.

 See references on p. 45.

Table 8 Commonly used antiemetics.

Antihistamines	e.g. cyclizine—for raised intracranial pressure and irritation of visceral and gastrointestinal serosa
Antidopaminergic agents	e.g. haloperidol, domperidone, methotrimeprazine, metoclopramide—for drug-induced, metabolic causes and anticipatory nausea
5HT antagonists	e.g. ondansetron—for chemotherapy-induced vomiting
Gastrokinetic	e.g. metoclopramide, domperidone —for delayed gastric emptying
Anticholinergic agents	e.g. hyoscine hydrobromide—for vestibular dysfunction
Mechanism of action uncertain	e.g. dexamethasone—for resistant nausea

5HT, 5-hydroxytryptamine.

2.4 Bowel obstruction

Aetiology

Bowel obstruction can occur at any site from the gastric outlet onwards. Patients with widespread intraperitoneal disease may have multiple sites of obstruction resulting from intraluminal deposits as well as external compression (Fig. 8).

Epidemiology

Bowel obstruction occurs in 10% of patients with colorectal carcinoma and 25% of those with carcinoma of the ovary.

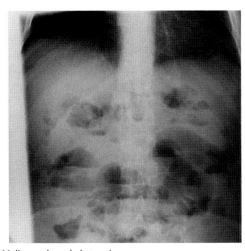

Fig. 8 Malignant bowel obstructions.

Treatment

 Do not neglect surgical options for palliation if the patient's wishes and general condition makes this appropriate.

Surgery

If the patient is fit, a colostomy or ileostomy can be performed. Ileostomy is indicated if there is a high obstruction or there are likely to be multiple sites of obstruction.

Corticosteroids

The role of steroids is unclear. Theoretically, they can reduce oedema around tumour deposits and thereby increase lumen size. Dexamethasone 12–16 mg s.c. or i.v. can be given for 7 days and then stopped if there is no improvement. Some patients improve considerably.

Octreotide

Obstructed bowel distends further as intraluminal secretions accumulate. A somatostatin analogue, octreotide, inhibits the release of hormones such as gastrin, secretin, vasoactive intestinal polypeptide (VIP) and pepsin among others. The inhibition of gastrointestinal secretions can break the cycle of distension and increased intraluminal secretions, thereby reducing vomiting and abdominal pain.

Antiemetics

Antiemetics may be ineffective or partially effective. Control of nausea and reduction of vomiting may be an achievable goal.

Analgesics

Subcutaneous diamorphine may control pain fully. If colic is present, use subcutaneous hyoscine butylbromide.

Nasogastric tubes

These may be occasionally required to relieve symptoms, but are unpleasant and other symptomatic measures should be tried first.

 See references on p. 45.
Mercadante S. The role of octreotide in palliative care. *J Pain Symptom Management* 1992; 7: 496.

2.5 Constipation

Aetiology

Common causes of constipation in patients with cancer are listed in Table 9.

Epidemiology

Constipation is defined as the passing of three or fewer stools per week. It is very common in the hospital population, affecting up to 63% of elderly patients and many with cancer.

Clinical presentation

Patients may present with abdominal pain, nausea and vomiting, or urinary retention. They may also present with agitation or confusion, or with spurious diarrhoea due to 'overflow'.

 It is important to take a good and detailed history of bowel actions as patients are often reticent to admit to problems of constipation.

 Prevention is better than cure—it is vital that constipation is treated prophylactically in patients starting opioids.

Table 9 Common causes of constipation in the cancer patient.

General	Debility
	Poor oral intake
	Confusion
	NHS loos/bed pans/lack of privacy
Drugs	Opioid drugs with anticholinergic effects, e.g. tricyclic antidepressants
	Diuretics
	Iron preparations
	Aluminium-based antacids
Malignancy	Lumbosacral cord, cauda equina or pelvic plexus damage
	Tumour within bowel
	Extrinsic compression of bowel by tumour
Local anal pathology	Haemorrhoids
	Anal fissure
	Bed sores
Other medical problems	Hypothyroidism
	Hypokalaemia
	Diabetes
	Diverticular disease

Physical signs

Faeces may be palpable either rectally or abdominally. Sometimes this is not obvious and an abdominal radiograph is needed to demonstrate faecal loading.

Treatment

Reversible causes should be treated and unnecessary medication stopped. Drug treatment may be necessary. Laxatives are either faecal softeners or stimulants. Combined preparations are available. The laxatives most commonly used are listed in Table 10.

Note that bulk laxatives do not have a place in the treatment of the seriously ill patient as they require a high-liquid intake and can be unpalatable.

 Case history example

A 73-year-old man with carcinoma of the prostate was started on morphine for bony pains. He was admitted to hospital with abdominal pain and diarrhoea. On questioning, he admitted that prior to the diarrhoea, he had not opened his bowels for 10 days. He had not been concerned as his appetite was poor and he therefore assumed he did not need to open his bowels. His rectum was clear. He was thought to have a high faecal impaction with overflow diarrhoea. Arachis oil and phosphate enemas were given with good effect. Normal bowel function was maintained with a combined stimulant/softener laxative.

 See references on p. 45.

Table 10 Types of laxatives used in patients with cancer.

Stimulants
These should be used for all patients starting opiates, unless there is malabsorption, e.g. ileostomy, pancreatic insufficiency. It is usual to give a faecal softener in addition. Commonly used stimulants are:
- bisacodyl
- senna
- sodium picosulphate

Softeners
- Docusate sodium (maximum 500 mg/day)
- Lactulose (maximum 15 mL twice daily)—this can cause bowel distension with increased abdominal cramps

Combined preparations
- Codanthramer—causes skin burns if incontinent
- Codanthrusate

Rectal preparations
Suppositories:
- glycerine—softening + mild stimulant
- bisacodyl—stimulant
Enemas:
- sodium citrate—stimulant
- phosphate—stimulant
- arachis oil—softener

2.6 Depression

Epidemiology

Depression is the most common psychiatric disease in patients with serious illnesses. The prevalence in the general population is 6–10%; figures quoted for patients with advanced cancer are 25–37%.

Patients at an increased risk are those with previous psychiatric problems, poor coping mechanisms and those who feel that communication about their illness—particularly during the 'bad news interview'—has not been appropriate for their needs.

Up to 80% of psychological and psychiatric morbidity in cancer patients goes undiagnosed.

Clinical presentation

Why is psychological and psychiatric morbidity undiagnosed in many patients with cancer? Is it due to:
• widespread acceptance of inevitability? ('of course they are depressed, they are dying!') or
• nurses' and doctors' sole concentration on physical symptoms?

Case history example

A 58-year-old man with recently diagnosed carcinoma of the bronchus attended clinic. He admitted to spending the whole day sitting watching television. He gained no pleasure from this and had difficulty in concentrating. His first long-awaited grandchild had just been born, but he expressed no desire to see her. He slept poorly, waking during the night, thinking about his disease and possible modes of death.

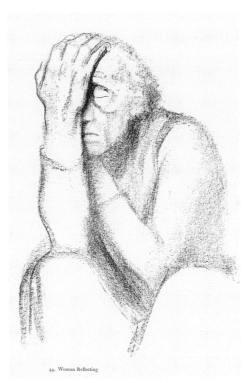

Fig. 9 Kathe Kollwitz: *Woman Reflecting.*

Table 11 Criteria for the diagnosis of depression in the healthy population.

1 Diminished interest or pleasure in all or almost all activities
2 Psychomotor retardation or agitation
3 Feelings of worthlessness or excessive and inappropriate guilt
4 Diminished ability to concentrate and think
5 Recurrent thoughts of death and suicide
6 Fatigue and loss of energy
7 Significant weight loss or gain
8 Insomnia or hypersomnia

There are no universally accepted criteria for diagnosing depression in the physically ill. In the physically healthy population, depression is diagnosed if patients have a persistent low mood and at least four of the symptoms listed in Table 11 are present most of the day for the preceding 2 weeks.

In patients with advanced cancer, symptoms 6–8 are almost universal. Endicott proposes that somatic symptoms should be substituted with the following:
• Diminished concentration—cannot be cheered up, does not smile, no response to good news or funny situation
• Fatigue and loss of energy—brooding, self-pity, pessimism
• Significant weight loss or gain—fearfulness or depressed appearance in body or face
• Insomnia or hypersomnia—social withdrawal or decreased talkativeness.

These are useful categories and much of the information needed to make a judgement as to whether the patient is depressed can be obtained by asking simple questions such as:
• 'how do you spend your day?'
• 'does any activity give you any pleasure?'
The doctor should not be afraid to ask about suicidal thoughts, perhaps using the question:
• 'do you have any thoughts of harming yourself?'
The patient will not be distressed; they will either refute it or show relief that someone has acknowledged the depth of their distress.

Treatment

The selective serotonin reuptake inhibitors (SSRIs) are generally well tolerated and are therefore gaining in popularity. Tricyclic antidepressants are also used for

41

neuropathic pain and are particularly useful when depression and pain coexist.

 Eighty per cent of patients with cancer and depression respond to antidepressants. It is therefore important to make the diagnosis and treat accordingly, even if their prognosis is weeks or months.

 Case history example

A 45-year-old maths teacher is admitted to the hospice. She had recently been told that her ovarian carcinoma had relapsed. She had taken to her bed, lying all day in a darkened room, refusing food or drink and saying she wanted to die. Her husband and children were distraught and unable to cope. She was eventually persuaded to see a liaison psychiatrist and to take antidepressants. Her mood improved after 3 weeks and she was discharged. She maintained a reasonably normal lifestyle for 3 months.

 See references on p. 45.
Lloyd-Williams M. The assessment of depression in palliative care patients. *Eur J Palliative Care* 1999; 6(5): 150–153.
Maguire P. Improving the detection of psychiatric problems in cancer patients. *Soc Sci Med* 1985; 20(8): 819–823.

2.7 Anxiety

Introduction

 Life's too short for worrying.
Yes, that's what worries me.
(Origin unknown)

Anxiety and difficulty in adjusting to a serious illness is common. Many patients will cope remarkably robustly with their problems; others will respond to reassurance, but some become increasingly incapacitated by anxiety. This can take many forms, often focusing on symptoms, possible mode of death, the family they are going to leave behind, and issues that are not resolved—'unfinished business'.

In many cases, anxiety is understandable:
• 'will my ex-husband, who left us 5 years ago, come and demand custody of the children?'
• 'we've been together for 50 years and we have no friends or family. He's never even boiled an egg.'

In other cases, the anxiety may be crippling in its intensity.

Clinical presentation

 Listen to the patient, seek guidance from their GP and the multidisciplinary team and treat accordingly.

The patient may declare their anxieties immediately, but many will not do so, thinking that 'they should not bother the doctor with them'. If you suspect anxiety, or things just don't add up, then ask—'I know that you must have many fears and worries, but is there anything in particular that is preying on your mind?'

Is treatment needed? Distinguishing anxiety which needs intervention from an expected level of distress or previous personality can be difficult. The patient often gives helpful information if you ask them to comment on their apparent anxiety, replying 'I've always been an anxious person', or 'this is not like me'.

Treatment

In many cases, anxiety responds well to simple non-pharmacological measures and patients can usually be maintained successfully at home under the care of their primary care teams. Psychologists offer help with coping strategies and counselling gives emotional support. Some patients are reassured by meeting others in similar situations at support groups or in hospitals.

Drug treatment

Benzodiazepines are the mainstay of treatment and can be given regularly or when needed. Sublingual lorazepam is effective for panic attacks.

 See references on p. 45.

2.8 Confusion

 'What is the answer?' After a short silence, she laughed and added 'Then what is the question?'
(Last words—Gertrude Stein, 1946)

Introduction

Acute confusional states are common in patients with advanced malignancy, increasing in prevalence as patients near their death. It is important to recognize confusion and to treat reversible causes. Confusion is distressing both for the patient, who may have lucid periods, and for the patient's relatives, who are often fearful and distressed.

The clinical approach to the patient with cancer who develops confusion is described in Section 1.4 (p. 30).

Investigation

Investigation of patients with advanced disease should be purposeful and kept to a minimum. The common treatable causes of confusion need to be excluded rapidly (see Table 1, p. 30). Ten to 20% of patients with solid tumours will become hypercalcaemic at some point in their disease.

Confusion without focal neurological signs is an uncommon presentation of cerebral metastases, but does sometimes occur. Investigate with an MRI/CT scan if the patient is fit enough to take high-dose corticosteroids and have palliative radiotherapy.

Include the relatives (and patient, if possible) when debating appropriate investigations. A calm and measured approach can do much to allay anxieties.

Treatment

Treat all reversible causes as rapidly as possible. You may feel that the patient is dying and that further antibiotics would be an unnecessary intrusion. Discuss this with the relatives, but do not imply to them that they are 'making the decision' (see *General clinical issues*, Section 3); they will rarely disagree with a clear and reasoned plan of care.

 Drugs may need to be stopped or opioids changed, e.g. morphine changed to hydromorphone or fentanyl.
Do not presume that morphine is always the cause of confusion. It is unlikely to be so if the patient has been on it without problems previously and renal function is stable.

Drug treatment for confusion is sometimes necessary and the following are suggested:
- Thioridazine 10–25 mg p.o. three times a day
- Haloperidol 2–5 mg p.o./s.c. three times a day
- Chlorpromazine 25–50 mg three times a day (very sedating).

 Confusion in elderly people—see *Medicine for the elderly*, Section 1.2.
A young woman who is ill and confused—see *Infectious diseases*, Section 1.2.
De Stoutz N. *Topics in Palliative Care*. New York: Oxford University Press, 1997.

2.9 The dying patient: terminal phase

 I'm not afraid to die, I just don't want to be there when it happens.
(Woody Allen, *Getting Even*)

Continuing careful management of the patient who is dying is important for the patient and their family. The aim of treatment is comfort for that patient and reduction of relatives' distress.

Common dilemmas

 Clear explanations to the patient and their relatives are needed.

Common dilemmas in management include:
- The use of antibiotics
- Intravenous hydration
- Sedation.

To tackle these and other issues you need to think of the following:
- Is the patient now inevitably dying of their disease?
- Would any intervention help symptoms?
- Would any treatment cause harm?

An approach based on these considerations should result in a treatment plan that is usually acceptable to the patient and their family. This may lead, for instance, to discontinuation of fluids in a patient who is not thirsty and remains comfortable with good mouth care. Conversely, you may prescribe antibiotics to a dying patient who is distressed by copious amounts of unpleasant bronchial secretions.

Clear explanations are needed, particularly about issues such as hydration, when the family will almost certainly need to be reassured that the patient is not dying because of dehydration, but because of their disease.

Symptom control

Symptoms need to be treated carefully. Different routes of administration may be needed when the patient has difficulty in swallowing.

If pain has been well controlled previously, it rarely becomes more difficult to manage in the terminal phase. Not all patients require or want sedation, and this should be discussed with them and their family. However, some become agitated or restless as death approaches, the causes of which are shown in Table 12.

Table 12 Causes of terminal agitation.

Physical	Pain
	Uncomfortable mouth
	Full bladder
	Full rectum
	'General stiffness'
	Inability to move
	Inability to communicate
Emotional	Fear of dying
	Distress on leaving family
	Unfinished business
Any cause of confusion	See Table 1, p. 30

Treatment

Terminal agitation and restlessness

The following are important:
- Continue analgesia and other drugs for symptom control
- Manage full bladder with catheterization
- Suppositories or enema may be necessary
- Calm nursing care
- Stop unnecessary treatments.

Drug treatments commonly used are shown in Table 13. A useful method of delivery for subcutaneous drugs is the syringe driver. The effect of stat doses can be used to determine the likely dose needed over 24 hours. As required doses (prn) should also be charted.

Case history example

A 56-year-old man with disseminated carcinoma of the bronchus was admitted to the hospice. He was dying but had become increasingly agitated. This had been interpreted as pain and his fentanyl had been changed to subcutaneous diamorphine and increased daily. On admission, he was on 15 g diamorphine per day, severely opiate toxic, agitated, twitching and hallucinating. Diamorphine was stopped completely and he was treated with midazolam and methotrimeprazine, of which large doses were needed. Once calm and comfortable, a small dose of diamorphine was restarted.

Terminal secretions

These are oral secretions accumulating in patients who are too weak to cough. They can be a cause of distress to relatives and the patient. Drug treatment includes the following.

Hyoscine hydrobromide

- Sedative, not to be used in the conscious patient.
- 400 µg every 4–6 hours or 400 µg to 2.4 mg over 24 hours via a syringe driver.

Glycopyrronium bromide

- Antimuscarinic and alternative to hyoscine.
- Fewer side effects and less sedating.
- 200 µg over 6 hours, maximum 800 µg/24 h via a syringe driver.

Kent. Vex not his ghost: O! Let him pass; he hates him
That would upon the rack of this tough world
Stretch him out longer.
(Shakespeare, *King Lear*)

See *General clinical issues*, Section 3
Higgs R. The diagnosis of dying. *J Roy Coll Physicians Lond* 1999; 2 March/April

2.10 Palliative care services in the community

Many patients wish to die at home, but despite this only around 29% do so. They are spending more of their last year of life at home but tend to die in institutions such as

Drug	Route of administration	Dose
Midazolam (anxiety and distress)	i.v., s.c., i.m.	10–60 mg/24 h
Methotrimeprazine (anxiety, distress, more sedating, antiemetic)	s.c., i.m., i.v., p.o.	12.5–250 mg/24 h
Haloperidol (also antiemetic)	s.c., i.v., i.m., p.o.	1.5–10 mg/24 h
Diazepam	p.o., p.r. (useful if rectal administration needed)	6–30 mg/24 h

Table 13 Drug treatment of terminal restlessness/agitation.

hospitals, hospices and nursing homes. There are several reasons for this:
- Patients may change their minds about care as death approaches
- Many feel that their illness is too great a burden for their relatives
- Lack of nursing care at home
- Worsening of symptoms
- Requests for hospital admissions from deputizing services or other GPs who are unfamiliar with the patient.

Inpatient units

There are inpatient palliative medicine units in all areas of the country. Some beds are NHS units attached to hospitals, while others are independent hospices funded by charities and health authorities.

Patients are admitted for symptom control, rehabilitation and terminal care: some units offer respite care for the benefit of patients and carers. Services may also include day care, outpatient clinics, lymphoedema treatment, acupuncture and alternative therapies. Staff should include specialists in palliative medicine, doctors in training, nurses, social workers, physiotherapists, occupational therapists and clergy, amongst others.

Emphasis is on improving quality of life and dealing with symptoms effectively so that patients can, if possible, be managed at home. Some units offer hospital at home or a sitting service.

Specialist palliative care nurses (sometimes called Macmillan nurses) provide advice on symptom control as well as psychological support. They form a link between the community and specialist palliative medicine units.

Hospital palliative care teams

These have palliative medicine consultants and specialist nurses as their core members. They advise hospital teams on symptom management and run the hospital palliative medicine service.

Marie Curie nurses

This service is for patients with advanced cancer and provides a maximum of 3 days' or nights' nursing care per week.

Ahmedzai S. *Oxford Textbook of Palliative Medicine*. New York: Oxford University Press, 1993.

Faull C, Carter Y, Wooff R. *Handbook of Palliative Care*. Oxford: Blackwell Science, 1998.

Higginson I. Where do cancer patients die? Ten year trends in the place of death of cancer patients in England. *Pall Med* 1998; 12: 353–363.

Hinton J. Can home care maintain an acceptable quality of life for patients with terminal cancer and their relatives? *Pall Med* 1994; 8: 183–196.

Final note

If possible, death should be peaceful (Fig. 10).

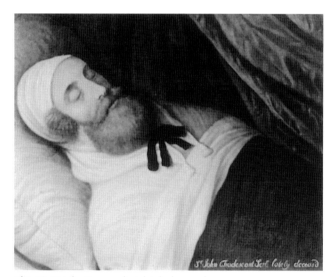

Fig. 10 St John Transcendant, lately deceased.

3 Self-assessment

Answers on pp. 101–102.

Question 1
A 78-year-old woman with carcinoma of the ovary is admitted with a 4-day history of constipation associated with colicky abdominal pain and vomiting. Which two of the following would you do?
A prescribe a laxative and paracetamol
B order a plain abdominal radiograph
C prescribe oramorph and metoclopramide
D arrange an abdominal ultrasound
E give a stat dose of diamorphine
F prescribe hyoscine butylbromide and cyclizine orally
G seek a surgical opinion
H insert a nasogastric tube
I start a syringe driver with diamorphine and metoclopramide
J start a syringe driver with diamorphine and cyclizine

Question 2
A 58-year-old woman with metastatic renal cancer presents with severe right leg pain radiating from her buttock to her toes. A recent CT scan demonstrates epidural invasion at L1–L4. The pain is described as sharp, tingling and she has altered sensations in her lower leg. There has been little response to 20 mg bd of morphine. What two initial approaches should be tried to control her pain?
A arrange radiotherapy
B titrate morphine dose
C give intravenous bisphosphonate
D arrange urgent intrathecal analgaesia
E add in paracetamol
F ask a counsellor to talk with her
G add in amitriptyline or gabapentin
H change to fentanyl patch
I refer back to oncologist for further chemotherapy
J set up diamorphine syringe driver

Question 3
A 78-year-old woman with carcinoma of the ovary is admitted with colicky abdominal pain and vomiting. A plain abdominal radiograph shows multiple fluid levels and no stool. She is on diamorphine in a syringe driver, but the pain persists. What would be your preferred two immediate options?
A give diamorphine prn
B add a fentanyl patch

C increase the dose of diamorphine in the syringe driver
D give a stat dose of midazolam
E add hyoscine hydrobromide
F insert a nasogastric tube
G give diazepam PR
H add hyoscine butylbromide to the syringe driver
I add midazolam to the syringe driver
J organise an abdominal ultrasound

Question 4
A 45-year-old man is dying from non-Hodgkin's lymphoma. He is increasingly agitated and distressed. He is not obviously in pain and has a urinary catheter in situ which is not causing specific distress. He has diamorphine 30 mg in his syringe driver. You are asked to review him. Select the best two options from the list below:
A increasing the diamorphine dose
B adding hyoscine hydrobromide
C no changes to his medication
D reducing the diamorphine dose
E adding midazolam 10 mg to the syringe driver
F giving a stat dose of midazolam
G changing diamorphine to fentanyl
H adding levomepromazine 75 mg to the syringe driver
I giving stat dose of levomepromazine 25 mg
J giving PR diazepam

Question 5
A 56-year-old man with metastatic carcinoma of the prostate has an epidural nerve block for neuropathic leg pain. Following this he is told to stop morphine sulphate continus (MST) but to take some oral morphine sulphate (Oramorph) should he develop any symptoms of opioid withdrawal. Two of these symptoms include:
A sweating
B abdominal pain
C dry mouth
D myalgia
E drowsiness
F cramps
G headache
H myoclonus
I hallucinations
J urinary retention

Question 6
A 40 year old man with complete spinal cord compression at T12 from bone metastases due to lung cancer has not

had his bowels open for 6 days. How would you best manage his symptom?

A avoid opioids and other constipating medicines

B prescribe high-dose co-danthramer

C perform rectal examination and prescribe high-dose co-danthramer

D prescribe and titrate polyethylene glycol until bowel movement

E perform PR with enema, prescribe low dose co-danthramer, then administer an enema 3 times per week

Question 7

You have decided to start a syringe driver on a dying patient whose symptoms were previously well controlled on oxycodone SR (OxyContin) 80 mg bd. What dose of diamorphine should you chose for your 24-hour syringe driver?

A 30 mg

B 60 mg

C 90 mg

D 110 mg

E 130 mg

Question 8

A 75-year-old woman with metastatic carcinoma of the colon is admitted semi-conscious and dying. Her symptoms had been previously well controlled on oxycodone SR 80 mg bd. What would you do about analgesia?

A nothing at present as she is semi-conscious and not obviously in pain.

B chart prn oxycodone orally

C change to im morphine

D chart prn paracetamol pr

E start a syringe driver with diamorphine

Question 9

A 69-year-old man with disseminated colon cancer is admitted with vomiting. You want to prescribe an antiemetic, but he is terrified that he might develop constipation, which has been a considerable problem for him in the past. Which one of the following anti-emetic drugs used in palliative care is not associated with constipation?

A ondansetron

B hyoscine

C cyclizine

D haloperidol

E levomepromazine

Question 10

A 50-year-old man with metastatic colorectal cancer complains of regurgitation of food and a feeling that it sticks retrosternally. Chest radiograph and upper gastrointestinal endoscopy are normal. Which antiemetic is most likely to be of benefit?

A cyclizine

B haloperidol

C prochlorperazine

D metoclopramide

E ondanestron

Question 11

A 54-year-old man with renal cell carcinoma and bone metastases is admitted with confusion and constipation. He is on morphine sulphate continus MST 100 mg bd and a non-steroidal anti-inflammatory drug. How would you manage him?

A avoid intrusive investigations and treat symptoms as they arise

B stop opiates which may be the cause of his symptoms

C reduce opiates

D change opiates

E check serum calcium

Question 12

A 58-year-old woman with carcinoma of the ovary has been taking morphine sulphate continus (MST) 200 mg bd for 3 months. She presents with a 2-day history of twitching and drowsiness. Examination reveals her to be fluid overloaded and have pin point pupils. What is the most likely cause of her symptoms?

A acute renal failure

B morphine overdose

C renal failure leading to accumulation of morphine

D brain secondaries

E right sided cardiac failure

Question 13

A frail 58-year-old woman with advanced breast cancer is admitted with abdominal pain and constipation secondary to opioids. Which of the following is the laxative of choice?

A sodium picosulphate

B ispaghula husk (Fybogel)

C senna

D co-danthramer

E lactulose

Question 14

A 58-year-old woman with metastatic carcinoma of the breast has good pain control on morphine sulphate continus MST 180mg bd. She is admitted with increasing weakness and has difficulty swallowing her tablets. It is therefore decided to convert her to a 24-hour diamorphine syringe driver. The correct dose of diamorphine is:

A 30 mg with 5 mg prn

B 60 mg with 10 mg prn

C 60 mg with 5 mg prn

D 120 mg with 10 mg prn
E 120 mg with 20 mg prn

Question 15

It has been decided that a patient should be changed from morphine sulphate continus MST 100 mg bd to the equivalent transdermal fentanyl dose. Choose the correct dose from those shown below:

A 125 μg/hr
B 25 μg/hr
C 100 μg/hr
D 50 μg/hr
E 75 μg/hr

Medicine for the Elderly

AUTHORS:
D. King, C.G. Nicholl & K.J. Wilson

EDITORS:
C.G. Nicholl & K.J. Wilson

EDITOR-IN-CHIEF:
J.D. Firth

1 Clinical presentations

1.1 Frequent falls

Case history

An 83-year-old retired headmistress presents after a fall. She falls frequently and is inclined to minimize the problem, but her health visitor daughter who lives about 100 km away is very concerned.

Clinical approach

Falls in older people are usually multifactorial. As described in Section 2.1 (p. 71), the effect of her diseases and drugs will interact with the background of ageing changes, loss of fitness and social factors. At 83 years, she is likely to have several coexisting diseases. The effects of normal ageing (e.g. increased sway) make falls more common with advancing years and potentially more serious (e.g. osteoporosis). Toddlers fall, but they are designed to! Sorting out falls requires a multidisciplinary, multiagency approach, and good communication with the patient and her family.

There are several important issues:
- What is causing the falls?
- What other factors may contribute?
- Have there been any serious consequences?
- Aim to prevent further falls, but, if this is not possible, minimize the consequences of falling.

History of the presenting problem

There may be clues in the history as to why she falls. Try to get a corroborative story from the patient's daughter (although she may not know), carers or GP. Specifically ask the following questions:
- How many falls have there been?
- Did she black out and for how long?
- Was she confused when she came round?
- Were there features of an epileptic fit?
- Did she feel dizzy? (cardiac/drugs)
- Any light-headedness, nausea and sweating? (syncope)
- Any palpitations? Intermittent atrial flutter/fibrillation is common and is not necessarily the cause of her falls (Fig. 1)
- What was she doing before the falls, e.g. standing up (postural hypotension), turning or reaching up for something (vertebrobasilar insufficiency)?
- Vertigo? (ear/brain-stem lesions)
- Do the falls occur outside (better prognosis as she is still able to get out) or in the home?
- What injuries have been sustained?
- Was she pushed? (elder abuse)

She may rationalize 'I must have tripped' when she has no idea what happened.

Relevant past history

Ask about the following:
- Strokes—CT brain scan showing multiple infarcts (Fig. 2)
- Epilepsy
- History of cognitive impairment
- Ischaemic heart disease
- Arthritis
- Previous fractures, thinking about osteoporosis.

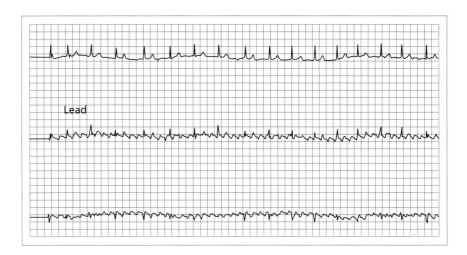
Fig. 1 ECG showing atrial flutter/fibrillation.

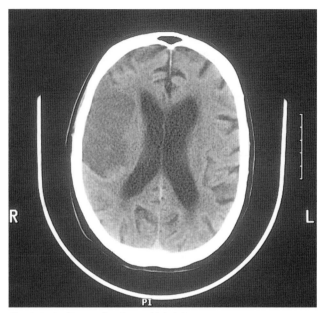

Fig. 2 Brain CT scan showing multiple infarcts.

Social history

Detailed information is essential:

• Does she live in a house with stairs, a bungalow (which may still have steps between rooms), sheltered accommodation or a residential home?
• Are there rails, bath aids, etc?
• Can she get out? (even in the UK, sunshine is the major source of vitamin D!)
• Alcohol?

 Alcoholism may be overlooked: 'but I've always drunk a few sherries, doctor, and it's never done me any harm'.

Occasionally, elderly people with no psychiatric illness live surrounded by all manner of junk in the 'senile squalor (Diogenes) syndrome'. It is hard not to trip.

Drug history

Older people are more susceptible to drug side effects, which may have more serious consequences. She is likely to be on several medications so interactions may occur.

 Remember to ask about over-the-counter (OTC) medication, e.g. decongestants are sedative.

Examination

• Is she ill, suggesting an acute condition, e.g. a silent myocardial infarct, pneumonia, a urinary tract infection (UTI) or hyponatraemia?

• Are there chronic, unrecognized problems, e.g. anaemia, hypo-/hyperthyroidism, cataracts?
• Has she been lying on the ground? (bruising, pressure sores, hypothermia)
• Are there any injuries?

Signs of neglect, such as poor personal hygiene or overgrown toenails, may point to dementia. In particular, check the following:

• General state, temperature, nutrition, mental test score
• Bones and joints, especially knees and hips, neck, 'spring' rib cage and pelvis
• Careful cardiological examination, including lying and standing blood pressure (BP) and carotid sinus massage
• Full neurological assessment looking for evidence of stroke, Parkinson's disease, myopathy or neuropathy
• Visual acuity
• Hearing and look for wax in the ears. If she has true vertigo, do the Hallpike manoeuvre to exclude benign paroxysmal positional vertigo
• Watch her walk. Look for a classic shuffling parkinsonian gait, a hemiplegic gait or the scissoring gait of a fixed arthritic pelvis. Watch her turn to assess balance
• Do not forget to look at her feet and shoes.

Consequences of this fall

Look for any complications of the fall:

• Soft-tissue injury: bruising, lacerations, burns
• Fractures: hip—most dangerous and requires prompt surgery and rehabilitation (see Section 2.8, p. 85); pelvis—needs admission and analgesia; sacral—painful but easily missed on radiograph; ribs—inadequate analgesia leads to pneumonia; wrist—may need admission if cannot manage activities of daily living or her walking frame
• Result of lying: pressure sores, incontinence.

Approach to investigations and management

Investigations

Be guided by the physical findings, but remember that some conditions may be 'silent' in elderly people:

• Full blood count: anaemia, macrocytosis of vitamin B_{12} deficiency, neutrophilia
• CRP: acute phase response to infection
• Urea and electrolytes, glucose: dehydration, hypo-/hyperglycaemia
• Creatinine kinase (CK): rhabdomyolysis is a risk after a long lie
• Liver profile: rise in alanine transaminase (ALT) for infarct is later than CK rise; may raise suspicion of alcoholism
• Bone profile: raised alkaline phosphatase (ALP) in vitamin D deficiency

- Thyroid function
- Midstream urine (MSU)
- ECG: rhythm, ischaemia, conduction defect
- 24-hour Holter monitor
- Chest radiograph: rib fractures, pneumonia, kyphosis suggesting osteoporosis

The following may also be appropriate:

- CT brain scan: vascular disease, space-occupying lesion, normal pressure hydrocephalus
- Electroencephalograph (EEG)
- Tilt-table testing.

> - Fear of falling leads to restriction of activity, which in turn leads to reduction of fitness and hence further falls.
> - Falls lead to pressure for institutionalization: the daughter who feels guilty as she lives at a distance insists that this would be safer, but falls happen in institutions! As a retired headmistress, this patient is used to being in control and wants to retain her independence.

Management

Once you have considered all the causes for her falls, identify those that are amenable to treatment:

- Treat specific diseases
- Stop/reduce dose of drugs that may contribute
- Manage other problems that increase risk of falls
- Improve general health and fitness (Tai Chi?)
- Treat osteoporosis in case she falls again
- Education and support (patient and her daughter): aim to reduce the likelihood of another fall and minimize the consequences if she does fall. A phone and duvet on the floor can be life saving! Try to educate the daughter to support her mother's right to take a risk and remain in her own home
- Specific information: provide contact numbers for patient-based societies, e.g. Parkinson's Disease Society, Stroke Association.

The multidisciplinary team has a key role in assessment and management (see Section 2.3, p. 74). The benefits of reducing the risks of further falls are the prevention of injuries, including fractures and therefore hospital admission, and also the promotion of the independence of elderly people in the community.

> Bandolier. *Falls in the Elderly* (1995) and *Injuries from Falls* (1999). Available at Bandolier home page, www.jr2.ox.ac.uk
> Gillespie LD, Gillespie WJ, Cumming R, Lamb SE, Rowe BH. Interventions for preventing falls in the elderly (Cochrane Review). In: *The Cochrane Library, Issue 3*, 2000. Oxford: Update Software.
> Lawson J, Fitzgerald J, Birchall J, Aldren CP, Kenny RA. Diagnosis of geriatric patients with severe dizziness. *J Am Geriatr Soc* 1999; 47: 12–17.
> Leaflets from Age Concern, RoSPA and patient societies.

1.2 Sudden onset of confusion

Case history

An 89-year-old woman is sent to the A&E department by a locum GP who was called when her evening carer found her wandering outside. The referral note states 'she is usually a bit muddled, but now cannot manage'. It is 2 a.m. and no other history is available.

Clinical approach

A diagnosis is essential for appropriate management. You need to decide whether she is confused or dysphasic.

> Fluent dysphasia in a stroke with little motor impairment often confuses the doctor.

If she is confused, is the confusion likely to be acute or chronic? The need for an evening carer suggests significant pre-existing physical or mental impairment. Can she tell you her name, age, the date or place? If you are not getting anywhere, check whether she can obey a one-step command that she would be able to perform physically, e.g. 'open your mouth'. She may be very deaf so use a communication aid, speak clearly with your face well lit or try writing. If you are still getting nowhere, examine her. Enlist a nurse, because you will need help.

> If she can give some answers, try short direct questions: 'are you in pain?' 'show me where' She may respond to your tone of voice and approach. Sound encouraging and don't appear to rush her; you may get more out of the history and examination.

Examination

Record her Abbreviated Mental Test (AMT) score (see Section 3.2, p. 94) and the Glasgow Coma Scale (GCS) (see *Emergency medicine*, Section 1.26). Observe nutritional state (reflects previous weeks to months) and hydration (reflects last 48 hours).

> Does her appearance suggest acute or chronic confusion? Well-presented clothing, clean styled hair, cleanliness and well-manicured toenails speak volumes—either this is an acute problem or you will have already met the carer!

A detailed examination is particularly important:
- in the absence of a good history

- because confusion has many causes
- as significant pre-existing pathology is likely.

This is not the time for short cuts.

 Don't be irritated—if she had been sent directly to a nursing home, the opportunity to treat any acute problem would have been missed. As well as the consequences for the individual, inappropriate admission to a home makes poor economic sense (Fig. 3).

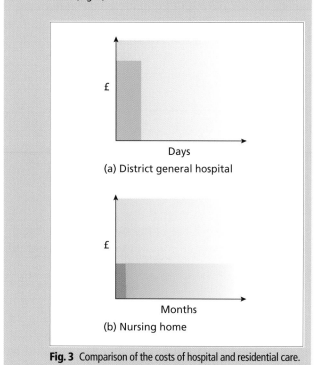

Fig. 3 Comparison of the costs of hospital and residential care.

(a) District general hospital

(b) Nursing home

Approach to investigations and management

There is a wide range of possible causes for an acute confusional state and these are listed in Table 1.

Investigations

These will depend on clinical features, but as non-specific presentation is common, tests marked with an asterisk are advisable in almost all patients.
- Full blood count*: low Hb and low mean corpuscular volume (MCV) suggest iron deficiency; high MCV suggests vitamin B_{12} or folate deficiency, hypothyroidism, alcoholism or myelodysplasia (predisposes to infection); neutrophilia suggests infection
- Urea, electrolytes and creatinine*
- Liver and bone profiles*: may need γ-glutamyltranspeptidase if alcohol is suspected or urgent calcium, e.g. if there is a history of breast cancer
- Cardiac enzymes*
- Glucose*
- Thyroid function*: thyroid-stimulating hormone (TSH) is the best screening test

- CRP*
- Blood cultures
- Syphilis serology: now rare in the UK; confusion with yaws in West Indian population; HIV serology if indicated
- Dipstick urine*: MSU or clean catch specimen may be difficult to obtain
- ECG*
- Chest radiograph*
- Oxygen saturation*: arterial blood gases in pneumonia or deranged acid–base balance
- Carboxyhaemoglobin
- Blood and urine for drug screen
- CT brain scan
- Lumbar puncture.

Management

 Management of her confusional state will depend on the results of investigations, but general principles apply: treat what you can now, try to prevent complications and obtain more information as soon as possible.

Immediate treatment

Balance the severity of her illness, her degree of confusion and what you need to achieve. A drip may be essential now to prevent prerenal failure (choose flat site of access and bandage very carefully). You may be able to give oral ciprofloxacin (excellent absorption), encourage cups of tea and drip 12 hours later when her confusion is settling but she is still behind on fluids. Remember the age and frailty of your patient—different antibiotics may be recommended in this age group (see Section 2.1, p. 71).

Preventive measures

Older patients often make a surprising recovery from the acute problem, only to linger in hospital with complications that could have been prevented:
- Is a better mattress needed to prevent pressure sores?
- Would subcutaneous heparin or compression stockings reduce the risk of deep venous thrombosis (DVT)?
- If she is incontinent, but you suspect a UTI, persuade the nurses that a catheter is not indicated until her constipation and the UTI have been treated, because a catheter will make any infection hard to clear.
- Is she safe? Are cot sides required? (If she keeps climbing over, talk over options such as leaving a light on, enlisting a relative, increasing the amount of nurse input or even putting the mattress on the floor.) Sedation may be necessary to enable her to have appropriate investigations or treatment, or if she appears distressed (risperidone 0.5 mg p.o. or haloperidol 0.5–2 mg i.m./p.o.).

Table 1 Causes of an acute confusional state.

Condition/mechanism		Example	Watch for
Intracranial pathology			
Vascular	Stroke	—	Frontal stroke with little paresis
Raised pressure	Space-occupying lesion	1°, 2°, subdural haematoma, abscess	Cerebral atrophy may minimize mass effect
Parkinson's disease	—		Subtle signs—the disease, its complications and treatment predispose to confusion
Epileptic fit	Postseizure or status		May present with focal signs too
Infection	Meningitis		Neck stiffness may be absent
	Encephalitis		Cranial herpes zoster with few skin lesions
Head injury	Concussion		Elder abuse is more common in confused individuals
Systemic pathology			
Infections	Chest, urine, cellulitis		Pyrexia absent or masked by mouth breathing
			Tachypnoea/cardia as the only signs of pneumonia
			SBE is less common but easily missed
Metabolic	Fluid, electrolyte or acid–base disturbance	Hyponatraemia	Drugs, e.g. thiazides, SSRIs, SIADH
		Hypernatraemia	Thirst may be blunted in elderly people
	Hypercalcaemia	Hyperparathyroidism	Check for mass in breast or thyroid
		Metastatic malignancy	Lymphadenopathy, 'invisible' surgical scars
		Excessive antacids	(neat healing in elderly people)
	Organ failure		Liver failure is usually obvious, uraemia less so
Endocrine	Diabetes	Hypoglycaemia	Prolonged with glibenclamide—not a drug of choice
		Hyperglycaemia	Elderly people may present with HONC
	Thyroid	Hypothyroidism	'Myxoedema madness'
		Hyperthyroidism	Confusion often exacerbated by AF
	Addison's disease		
Shock/hypoxia	Pump failure	MI	Chest pain may be absent. Mechanism may be hypotension, LVF or both
		Tachy- or bradydysrhythmias	Always exclude hyperthyroidism in fast AF
	Respiratory failure	COPD, end-stage fibrosis	In severe COPD, give nebulizers with air
	Loss of blood volume	Gastrointestinal bleed, bleed into a hip fracture	Usually apparent, but melaena may be delayed in severe constipation
			Warfarin, NSAIDs and aspirin are common drugs
	Loss of vascular tone		Overwhelming sepsis, e.g. intra-abdominal emergency: perforation, obstruction (check for femoral hernia), mesenteric ischaemia (acidosis and high K$^+$)
	Severe anaemia		Usually chronic
	Carbon monoxide poisoning		Husband and wife may present together
Nutritional deficiencies		Wernicke's encephalopathy (thiamine deficiency)	Other deficiencies, e.g. of nicotinic acid and vitamin B$_{12}$, tend to present as chronic confusion
Hypothermia			Check rectal temperature with low-reading thermometer
Unreported discomfort	Hip or pelvic fracture		Missed in agitated confused patients with other pathology, e.g. a stroke
	Faecal impaction		Rectal examination is essential
Drugs and withdrawal			Prescribed and OTC drugs
			Accidental or intentional overdose
Alcohol and withdrawal			A few days illness may have prevented the usual intake of alcohol

AF, atrial fibrillation; COPD, chronic obstructive pulmonary disease; HONC, hyperosmolar non-ketotic coma; LVF, left ventricular failure; MI, myocardial infarct; NSAID, non-steroidal anti-inflammatory drug; OTC, over the counter; SBE, subacute bacterial endocarditis; SIADH, syndrome of inappropriate secretion of antidiuretic hormone; SSRI, specific serotonin reuptake inhibitor.

The next morning

Back to the history! You need to know what she was like before the problem that precipitated admission. Time on the phone is time well spent. Her own GP will know her drugs and past history and may know about her mental state. If her carer is regular, she will be able to describe her usual capabilities (dressing, transfers, walking, continence), her short- and long-term memory, orientation (does she recognize the carer or get lost about the flat?) and how she occupies her day. What changed and over what period of time? Before things went wrong, was the home situation adequate or have things been deteriorating for a while? Is everyone (except possibly the patient) declaring that 'a home' is essential?

> Identify key players in the community (professionals, family, friends and informal carers) at an early stage. Will distant relatives—the nephew who is an orthopaedic surgeon in New York—suddenly materialize with their own views?

A common situation

The most common diagnoses would be an acute confusional state caused by a chest or urinary tract infection or medication, superimposed on a background of moderate dementia, usually Alzheimer's disease [2,3] (see Section 2.7, p. 83). When her acute confusion has resolved, evaluate her mood. Treating unrelated but compounding pathology, e.g. cataracts, can produce dramatic improvement.

> You need to think ahead as patients like this can get stuck in the hospital system. Minimize potential delays by early referrals to occupational therapy, physiotherapy, dietetics and social services.

Planning discharge

This will be time-consuming if she has significant dementia, but is sure she can manage. In the UK, it is rare for old people with dementia to be sectioned under the Mental Health Act. Despite the risk of failure, discharge with a maximal care package is usually arranged. A home visit followed by a case conference with members from the community health team may be needed to optimize the package. Phone the GP before the discharge.

> If the home situation is very borderline, the patient's wishes and determination are crucial. Some members of the team and the family may feel that 'it is a disgrace to allow her to return to such squalor!' Try not to impose standards on others—she has survived for 89 years and is a 'nice residential home' really a better prospect?

Other suggestions for management of dementia are given in Section 2.7, p. 83.

1 McKeith IG, Perry EK, Perry RH. Report of the Second Dementia with Lewy Body International Workshop: diagnosis and treatment. Consortium on Dementia with Lewy Bodies. *Neurology* 1999; 53: 902–905.
2 Small GW, Rabins PV, Barry PP *et al.* Diagnosis and treatment of Alzheimer disease and related disorders. Consensus statement of the American Association for Geriatric Psychiatry, the Alzheimer's Association, and the American Geriatrics Society. *JAMA* 1997; 278: 1363–1371.
3 Morris JC. Alzheimer's disease: a review of clinical assessment and management issues. *Geriatrics* 1997; 52(suppl 2): S22–S25.
4 Thurston JG. Management of acute confusion in the elderly. *Eur J Emerg Med* 1997; 4: 103–106.

1.3 Urinary incontinence and immobility

Case history

A 79-year-old housewife has been referred with urinary incontinence and decreasing mobility over the past 18 months. The letter from the GP makes it clear that the home situation is breaking down. She has great difficulty reaching the toilet in time. Her only medication is one co-amilofruse tablet.

Clinical approach

First, consider the two problems separately, although one diagnosis could explain both, e.g. incontinence is an early finding in normal pressure hydrocephalus (NPH) and Parkinson's disease is a cause of urge incontinence.

> Chronic disease may be undetected in elderly people because both they and their carers accept problems such as poor mobility, deteriorating memory and incontinence as a normal part of ageing. It is only when the family can no longer cope that medical advice is sought.

Differential diagnosis of poor mobility

This could be caused by a wide range of problems:
• Neurological: stroke, Parkinson's disease, NPH, cerebellar disease, cord lesion and neuropathies
• Musculoskeletal: all types of arthritis, myopathy, painful feet
• Psychiatric: depression, dementia
• Cardiorespiratory: severe cardiac failure, angina, peripheral vascular disease or chronic lung disease
• Morbid obesity.

History of the presenting problem

The major system limiting mobility will usually be clear: neurological, musculoskeletal or psychiatric.

Neurological

• Onset of symptoms: sudden with cerebrovascular accident (CVA), gradual with Parkinson's disease, step-wise with multi-infarct dementia
• Symptoms of Parkinson's disease: difficulty turning over in bed, freezing, dribbling.

Musculoskeletal

• Joint pains associated with joint swelling and early morning stiffness in rheumatoid arthritis
• Pain, deformity and crepitus in knees and hips suggestive of osteoarthritis
• Difficulty rising from a chair suggestive of proximal myopathy, e.g. thyrotoxicosis and vitamin D deficiency, or muscle discomfort, e.g. polymyalgia or polymyositis
• Bone pain (see Section 1.6, p. 63).

Psychiatric

• Loss of appetite, insomnia, poor concentration and anhedonia of depression
• Poor memory, confusion and disorientation of acute or chronic confusion.

Whatever the main cause, a number of factors may contribute and a vicious cycle may have developed so that loss of fitness may be a major component.

Examination

Look for the features of the diseases listed above and watch the patient rise from a chair, walk and turn.
• Mask facies, pill-rolling tremor, cogwheel rigidity, loss of arm swing, flexed posture and shuffling gait (Parkinson's disease)
• Broad-based gait or gait apraxia and confusion (NPH)
• Hemiplegia
• Examine joints for evidence of acute or long-standing arthritis
• Record an AMT score and Geriatric Depression Score (GDS) (see Section 3.2, pp. 94–95).

Approach to investigations and management

Investigations

These will be dictated by clinical findings but often include a CT brain scan and radiographs of affected joints.

Management

This patient was found to have Parkinson's disease and was referred to the specialist clinic for multidisciplinary assessment. Options for management include the following:
• Drug treatment—probably levodopa with peripheral decarboxylase inhibitor in this case (see Neurology, Section 2.3)
• Education, advice and support to patient and carer from nurse specialist
• Gait practise, exercise and balance work, and assessment for aids by the physiotherapist (Rollators usually preferred to Zimmer frames which turn walking into a sequence of stops and starts—not ideal in Parkinson's disease)
• Assessment of the patient and her home by the occupational therapist
• Speech and language therapy (swallowing, facial expression and speech)
• Social worker who will assess for benefits (see Section 2.12, p. 91) and will tailor a package of care around each patient's needs
• Organizations such as the Parkinson's Disease Society are an excellent source of information for patients, carers and doctors!

Differential diagnosis of incontinence

There are several types of incontinence which are managed differently, so a correct diagnosis is essential.

 Distinguish between urge, stress and overflow incontinence or a mixed picture.

History of the presenting problem

The history usually helps determine the probable cause, so ask the patient to keep a continence diary, recording times and volumes of voiding and any accidents. Ask specifically:
• Does she have a frequent, sudden, overwhelming desire to pass urine, often not reaching the toilet in time? Does she have to pass urine frequently during the night? (urge incontinence)
• Does she pass small amounts of urine on coughing, laughing or exercising? (stress incontinence)
• Does she have dysuria and frequency? (urinary tract infection)
• Is she constipated?
• Ask men about poor stream, dribbling and nocturia suggestive of prostatism.

	Bladder irritation	Sedative effect	Urinary retention	Diuretic effect	Relaxation of prostatic smooth muscle
Alcohol	✓	✓	—	✓	—
Caffeine	✓	—	—	✓	—
Antipsychotic medication (e.g. chlorpromazine)	—	✓	✓	—	—
Antidepressants (e.g. lofepramine)	—	✓	✓	—	—
Benzodiazepines (e.g. diazepam)	—	✓	—	—	—
α-blockers (e.g. doxazosin)	—	—	—	—	✓
Diuretics (e.g. furosemide (frusemide))	—	—	—	✓	—

Table 2 Drugs increasing the risk of incontinence.

Relevant past history

Social history

Ask about the number and size of babies and trauma to the perineum, and any pelvic surgery, particularly hysterectomy and oophorectomy. Symptoms such as vaginal dryness and dyspareunia correlate better with atrophic vaginitis than mucosal appearance.

Drug history

Remember that alcohol, caffeine and aspartame all irritate the bladder (Table 2). Check her list of drugs, especially diuretics, anticholinergic drugs and sedatives.

Examination

The examination focuses on the abdomen, but the legs must also be examined neurologically. In the abdomen check the following:
• Is the bladder palpable? Are there any pelvic masses, e.g. ovarian tumours pressing on the bladder?
• Rectal examination: faecal loading, anal tone and perineal sensation, and prostatic size and nature in men
• Vaginal examination: prolapse, cystocele
• Stress test: does she leak urine on coughing?

Approach to investigations and management

Investigations

• Urine dipstick: if there are nitrites or leucocytes, send an MSU. Haematuria needs renal tract ultrasonography and urology assessment.
• Ultrasonography: assess chronic retention and residual volume.
• Urodynamic studies are indicated if there is no improvement in her symptoms after simple interventions (see Section 2.4, p. 78).

Management

 The secret of success is early liaison with the hospital or community continence adviser.

• Stop any unnecessary drugs that may contribute.
• Try regular toileting and bladder retraining.
• Improvement in her mobility will help.
• This patient has symptoms of urgency. She would benefit from a trial of anticholinergic therapy: oxybutynin or tolterodine. Starting with the lowest dose reduces the risk of side effects such as confusion.
• If she had symptoms and signs of stress incontinence, encourage pelvic floor exercises first. If there is no improvement and she is fit for surgery, refer to a uro-gynaecologist for bladder neck surgery.
• If all of the above fail, consider pad and pants, or an indwelling catheter.

This patient responded well to co-careldopa (Sinemet) and the input from the Parkinson's disease team. Management of her incontinence involved several lines of treatment. Stopping her diuretic (prescribed inappropriately for dependent oedema), treating her UTI and chronic constipation, and a bladder training regimen made a great difference, particularly as her mobility improved. Treating mild anaemia caused by dietary folate and iron deficiency improved her well-being, but the greatest difference was achieved by referring her for cataract surgery. Two years later she continues to manage at home, with a home help twice a week.

 Continence Society website: http://www.vois.org.uk/cf
Dawson C, Whitfield H. Urinary incontinence and urinary infection. *BMJ* 1996; 312: 961–964.
Parkinson's Disease Society website: http://glaxocentre.merseyside.org/pds.html
Rosenthal AJ, McMurtry CT. Urinary incontinence in the elderly. *Postgrad Med* 1995; 97: 109–121.

1.4 Collapse

Case history

An 84-year-old retired gardener presents to A&E. The previous evening he got up to pass water and slumped to the floor. His wife got him back to bed, but this morning he was drowsy and not moving his right side.

Clinical approach

Initial rapid assessment is required. While checking his vital signs and glucose, you notice facial asymmetry and a hemiparesis.

History of the presenting problem

Take the history from his wife on a stroke proforma if used locally. She will be upset and may need sympathetic prompting (see *Neurology*, Section 2.8.1).

Look for:
- Features that raise the likelihood that this is not a stroke (progressive disability).
- Pointers to a rare cause of stroke such as arteritis.
- Any event preceding the collapse (e.g. chest pain or melaena (hypotension), head injury or a fit and Todd's paresis).

Drugs are a useful prompt: 'was enalapril for blood pressure or swollen ankles?' Family history is less relevant than in a young patient, but you may get information about his wife's experience of stroke. Record his past history, forming an impression of disease burden. In the social history, note information about accommodation, family and other support, but if he survives this will need to be revisited in detail. Touch on his lifestyle and interests. Meanwhile, will his wife manage or will she need support at home?

Examination

A full examination is needed, but in particular:
- confirm your diagnosis
- determine his conscious level (Glasgow Coma Score) and the extent of the neurological impairment
- check for early complications, e.g. aspiration pneumonia, erythematous heels
- identify risk factors for secondary prevention (limited evidence at this age, but sensible management of hypertension, atrial fibrillation, diabetes)
- document major co-morbidities.

When you talk to his wife, it may be easier to broach the subject of what he would have wanted if things do not go well at this stage, rather than 'cold' a couple of days later. If he had made a living will (see Section 2.13, p. 93), this gives her the opportunity to mention it. In the event of cardiac arrest, resuscitation is most unlikely to succeed, so explain that, although you are going to do everything for him, should he collapse unexpectedly you will keep him comfortable.

Approach to investigations and management

Investigations

Full blood count (FBC), electrolytes and renal function, biochemical profile, CRP, glucose, TSH, chest radiograph, ECG, pulse oximetry, CT brain scan; and other tests if indicated.

Management

Immediate management

There is now clear evidence [1] that the patient should be managed on a stroke unit but, whatever the setting, pay attention to the following:
- Pressure area care; the worst damage is often done on the A&E trolley
- Compression stockings; subcutaneous heparin is not indicated
- Conveen if possible rather than catheter
- Antibiotics to cover aspiration if there are chest signs
- Rectal paracetamol if febrile
- Which regular drugs need to be continued? (a nasogastric tube may be needed if no parenteral option, e.g. levodopa)
- Antihypertensive drugs are not indicated for acute hypertension
- If drowsy or unable to sit, intravenous fluids and nil by mouth; if alert and able to sit, observe drinking sips, and then 50 mL water
- Correct positioning to minimize spasticity and avoid complications such as subluxation at a flaccid shoulder.

Within 24 hours

Unless the patient is moribund, active management is required to prevent complications:
- Early physiotherapy—chest and passive movements
- Aspirin if CT excludes haemorrhage
- If there is doubt about safe swallow, request speech and language therapy assessment. Thick yoghurt is usually the texture swallowed most safely so thickening agents are often recommended; thin fluid with bits, e.g.

minestrone soup, is the most challenging! The patient should always be sitting upright before having food. If in doubt continue nil by mouth.

The next few days

• Reassess swallowing daily. Weigh as soon as possible. Within a few days, if the patient still cannot swallow but is not dying, consider a fine-bore nasogastric (NG) tube taped to the paralysed side to allow feeding and maintain hydration. If there is doubt, arrange videofluroscopy to check for pooling or aspiration.
• Help the relatives—having nerved themselves for his death, this hasn't happened but the situation looks grim. Encourage his wife to eat, take breaks and pace her visits. Explain that, although sudden deterioration is possible (further stroke, myocardial infarction or pulmonary embolism), bronchopneumonia is more likely. Provide literature from the Stroke Association [2] about stroke and relevant complications, e.g. dysphasia.
• Refer to speech and language therapy for communication assessment. If he is drowsy or dysphasic, early assessment may help the family and staff to communicate, e.g. he may master a picture chart.
• When his condition permits, start speech therapy and active physiotherapy. He should spend time nursed well positioned in a chair with adequate pressure relief (drowsiness, cognition and trunk control permitting).

After 1–2 weeks

If he still cannot swallow, but overall things are improving, consider referral for percutaneous endoscopic gastrostomy (PEG) feeding. PEG feeding permits better nutrition (NG tubes usually fall out regularly) and more dignity, but does not remove the risk of aspiration. Paradoxically, in some situations, an advantage of NG tubes is that they do fall out—it is easier not to resite a tube than it is to remove one. If he is deteriorating or the swallow is improving, persevere with NG feeding. In a patient with severe dementia who reaches for food or drink despite a tendency to choke, a policy of nil by mouth and PEG is unkind, and supervised oral feeding with thickening agents is appropriate.

 A PEG tube is not always advisable and should be inserted only after multidisciplinary discussion involving the family, especially if the patient cannot understand the procedure.

Allowing the patient to die

Advice is available in the BMA guidelines [3]. Patients who are going to die usually do, but death may be prolonged by medical intervention. Defer a CT brain scan rather than risk the patient dying in the scanner. In end-stage dementia, antibiotics may be inappropriate from the start. Usually, the situation is less clear and most patients with a severe stroke will receive antibiotics for their first infective complication.

If, 2 or 3 weeks later, there is no useful recovery and the patient is chesty, is it time to let nature take its course? By now you may have a feel for what the patient wanted and the family view, 'he was such an independent, outdoor man …'. Don't place the burden of decision on the family. A medical decision, taking account of the view of the multidisciplinary team in the interests of the patient, is needed. This should then be discussed with the family. If there is disagreement, remember that many doctors and most of the public have an inflated view of the power of antibiotics.

 It often helps to explain that: 'treatment with antibiotics usually works only with other measures such as physiotherapy to clear his chest. Physiotherapy will not be very effective because he cannot work with the therapist, and it may be uncomfortable or distressing (suction) for him, as we cannot explain to him what we are trying to do. As a result of the severe brain damage, even if we can get him through this infection, he is likely to get another soon.'

Given a full explanation, families usually agree with keeping comfortable an elderly patient with a massive stroke.

 Check that all significant family members agree. If the family is not ready to accept palliation, consider further antibiotics to give them more time. A second opinion may be useful.

If the patient is dying, ensure that symptom control is optimal, as in patients dying from cancer (see *Palliative care*, Section 3.1).

Rehabilitation

PREPARING FOR REHABILITATION

If he pulls through, treat other problems pragmatically. He used to take an NSAID for his arthritic knees. Adequate analgesia is essential if he is to mobilize, but regular paracetamol is usually effective. You have noted iron deficiency anaemia. Surgery would not be indicated so do not put him through the investigations. Oesophagitis or peptic ulceration is possible, so prescribe a proton pump inhibitor and recheck his FBC in 2 weeks. As he progresses, look for opportunities to improve things, e.g. replace lost spectacles. If he deteriorates, find out why (constipation, UTI, further stroke).

SLOW STREAM REHABILITATION

Rehabilitation after a major stroke is a long haul. The setting will depend on what is available locally. There is no clear advantage for early supported discharge schemes, although they may free hospital capacity [4] (see Section 2.8, p. 85).

The patient's co-morbidites, previous fitness, cognition and mood, and the attitude of the family determine what may be achieved with a given level of neurological impairment. In outline, the contributions of the multidisciplinary team are:
- the physiotherapist will work on posture, balance and functional movement. Appliances, such as a wrist or ankle splint, may be helpful
- the occupational therapist will assess basic activities of daily living (personal ADLs), then more sophisticated abilities (instrumental or IADLs), to promote independence
- the speech and language therapist will work on communication and swallowing
- the social worker may advise on benefits and will help plan placement
- the dietitian and, in rare units, a psychologist, art or music therapist may be involved
- a Stroke Association volunteer may come in from the community
- the doctor will be involved with on-going and new medical problems
- the nursing staff are the key people in the team. Their skill in ensuring that the patient is in a co-ordinated therapeutic environment all day, rather than for a couple of brief therapy sessions, is crucial.

Progress is monitored against explicit goals agreed with the patient and family, and new goals are set at regular (often weekly) multidisciplinary case conferences. If the patient is not making the expected progress, can a barrier to rehabilitation be identified (e.g. depression or the fear of being a burden)? Complications of stroke such as emotional lability, personality change or cognitive impairment, difficulties with bowels and bladder, and poststroke pain may benefit from a team approach.

Placement

The focus shifts from rehabilitation to placement once the patient's gain from therapy reaches a plateau. The timing depends on how much rehabilitation can be provided in the community.

 Plan early (e.g. home visit from an occupational therapist) for the likely destination—change tack later if necessary. Don't defer to see what the patient achieves because there will then be a frustrating wait while support is arranged.

Common options are home with a support package, rehousing to a warden-supervised flat, a residential home, nursing home or, in a few areas, NHS nursing care. Your assessment must take account of the carer's needs. Consider regular respite or a service such as Crossroads, which will offer a regular sitter to allow the carer a break.

Funding of long-term care is a political hot potato because of the huge cost. Patients with major disabilities can go home—usually if accommodation needs little adaptation—to a willing able-bodied carer, but the time to assemble the necessary equipment, e.g. hospital bed, pressure mattress, standing hoist, appropriate wheelchair, etc., can be lengthy. The carer should work alongside therapists before discharge. A sensible spouse can manage a PEG tube—sterility is not needed but training is essential.

Reassessment should be planned because unexpected problems will arise and, after the initial elation at discharge, depression may resurface. The patient may attend the day hospital before and after discharge to provide continuity of care.

 Good start point for surfing: http://www.dundee.ac.uk/ medicine/Stroke/index.htm
1 Gubitz G, Sandercock P. Extracts from 'Clinical Evidence': acute ischaemic stroke. *BMJ* 2000; 320: 692–696.
2 Stroke Association website: http://www.stroke.org.uk
3 British Medical Association. *Withholding and Withdrawing Life-prolonging Medical Treatment: Guidance for Decision Making*. London: BMJ Books, 1999.
4 Early Supported Discharge Trialists. Services for reducing duration of hospital care for acute stroke patients (Cochrane Review). In: *The Cochrane Library, Issue 3*, 1999. Oxford: Update Software.

1.5 Vague aches and pains

Case history

A 79-year-old retired tax man is referred with a 1-month history of sudden onset but vague aches and pains, weight loss and general malaise. He takes glipizide for type 2 diabetes, atorvastatin for raised cholesterol and ibuprofen for back pain secondary to 'wear and tear'. Routine blood tests show a normocytic anaemia with a haemoglobin of 10.9 g/dL, normal urea and electrolytes, and an ESR of 95 mm/h.

Clinical approach

A comprehensive assessment is required.

 Malaise with a high ESR is a very common scenario. The important differential diagnoses are:
- polymyalgia rheumatica (PMR)/giant cell arteritis (GCA) (see *Rheumatology*, Section 2.5.1 and *Ophthalmology*, Section 2.6) [1,2]
- myeloma (is the back pain more sinister?)
- late-onset rheumatoid arthritis
- carcinoma of the prostate and colon, and other malignancies
- osteoarthritis, especially cervical spondylosis with another cause for a raised ESR
- depression with another cause for a raised ESR
- lymphoma or low-grade leukaemia
- polymyositis, including drug-induced
- poorly controlled diabetes, which with a chronic infection and neuropathy could present a similar picture.

History of presenting complaint

 The risk of blindness makes GCA a diagnosis not to miss.

Check the following:
- Any change in vision, reduced acuity or diplopia?
- Pain in the jaw when chewing?
- Tenderness of the scalp when combing the hair?
- Influenza-like symptoms? (there may be a prodromal illness in PMR or GCA)
- Early morning stiffness?
- Change in bowel habit, blood in the stools?
- Symptoms of depression?
- When was his atorvastatin prescribed? (myositis is a rare but significant side effect of statins)

Examination

 Many elderly patients investigated for 'weight loss' weighed more in middle age, but have been a stable weight for several years.

Remember to check for the following:
- Objective evidence of weight loss (weigh now and look back at clinic or inpatient weights)
- Low-grade fever (common in PMR)
- Scalp tenderness
- Inflammation of the temporal arteries: thickening, nodularity, loss of pulsatility or tenderness
- Lymphadenopathy
- Abdominal examination, including rectal examination, looking for masses and hepatomegaly
- Muscle tenderness
- Examine all of his joints; can he raise his arms above his head?
- Visual acuity and fundoscopy (looking for arteritis and diabetic retinopathy) (see *Ophthalmology*, Sections 2.6 and 2.7)
- Other complications of his diabetes.

Approach to investigations and management

Investigations

Depending on the picture consider:
- CRP and repeat ESR
- FBC and film
- liver and bone biochemistry (hepatic ALP is often raised in GCA)
- muscle CK
- rheumatoid factor
- glycosylated haemoglobin, to check diabetic control
- prostate-specific antigen and radiograph of lumbar spine
- myeloma screen: immunoglobulins, Bence-Jones urinary proteins, skeletal survey
- radiographs of joints as indicated by examination
- chest radiograph
- abdominal CT scan or barium enema or colonoscopy
- temporal artery biopsy; there is debate as to whether this is indicated in PMR. A positive result confirms the diagnosis, but a negative result does not exclude it. Do not delay steroid treatment if GCA is a possibility—if a biopsy is going to be positive, it still will be after a 'few' (controversy in the literature) days on treatment
- electromyograph (EMG) or nerve conduction studies if myositis or neuropathy is suspected.

Management

This patient had no signs of cranial arteritis and his temporal artery biopsy was negative. He was not depressed. His CK was normal, so myositis associated with his atorvastatin was not likely, but this could be stopped (need to review cardiovascular risk factors, consider his biological age and make a clinical judgement in the absence of trial data at this age). In view of his symptoms of pain and stiffness, he was diagnosed as having PMR. Treatment was with steroids, but there are no good prospective trials to give clear information about the dose and duration of treatment.

He was told to report any visual symptoms at once and commence prednisolone 15–20 mg daily for 1 month. This is much lower than the dose that is essential for treating GCA. His ibuprofen was replaced with regular paracetamol since the risk of gastrointestinal bleeding using an NSAID with steroids in this age group is high.

 If the diagnosis is PMR, the symptoms of malaise and stiffness will melt away 'like magic' in 2–3 days on 20 mg prednisolone. If this does not occur, reconsider your diagnosis. The clinical response is more useful than a fall in CRP or ESR, because these usually fall on administration of steroids, whatever the underlying condition.

The prednisolone dose should be reduced by 2.5 mg every 2–4 weeks until the dose is 10 mg, then by 1 mg every 4–6 weeks guided mainly by the patient's symptoms. Most patients require treatment for 3–4 years, but a third to a half may be able to stop after 2 years. Try to stop steroids at this point and watch for relapse.

Important points about steroid use

 Steroid treatment causes serious morbidity and mortality in elderly people.

• Particularly because of the clinical nature of the diagnosis of polymyalgia, it is often difficult weaning patients off their steroids.
• Give bone prophylaxis with a bisphosphonate or calcium and vitamin D (e.g. Calceos) if bisphosphonates are poorly tolerated or the patient is house-bound.
• He is frail, anaemic and has been on ibuprofen, so even in the absence of a history of peptic ulcer (often silent) gastric protection with an H_2-receptor blocker or proton pump inhibitor is advisable.
• The hyperglycaemic action of prednisolone is likely to impair his diabetic control, which should be monitored carefully.
• Fluid retention may precipitate cardiac failure (increased risk because of his diabetes, possible heart disease as indicated by his hypercholesterolaemia and NSAID).
• Steroid psychosis can be problematic, although usually at higher doses.
• Elderly people are more susceptible to all of the side effects of steroids (those above, plus increased susceptibility to infection, weight gain, masking of perforated viscus, etc.) and there is a case for using steroid-sparing drugs, such as azathioprine or methotrexate.
• The steroid dose should be increased during periods of stress, e.g. severe illness and perioperatively.

 1 Pountain G, Hazelman B. Polymyalgia rheumatica and giant cell arteritis. *BMJ* 1995; 310: 1057–1059.
2 Swanell AJ. Polymyalgia rheumatica and temporal arteritis: diagnosis and management. *BMJ* 1997; 314: 1329–1332.

1.6 Swollen legs and back pain

Case history

A 79-year-old man complains of severe lower backache, fatigue and leg swelling which has caused decreased mobility for 6 weeks. He has lived alone all his life and had only occasionally consulted his GP for respiratory tract infections in the winter months.

Clinical approach

A full clinical history and examination are essential, but you will focus on finding the cause of the swelling and back pain.

 Causes of peripheral oedema

• Gravitational as a result of immobility—a common cause in elderly people.
• Side effects of drugs causing fluid retention, e.g. steroids, NSAIDs and fludrocortisone, or vasodilatation, e.g. calcium channel blocker or, in hospital, intravenous fluids.
• Congestive heart failure.
• Hypoalbuminaemia resulting from undernutrition.
• Chronic venous insufficiency.
• Venous obstruction caused by thrombosis or external compression by pelvic malignant disease.
• Lymphatic obstruction.
• Nephrotic syndrome, chronic renal failure.
• Chronic liver disease.

 Causes of lower backache

• Lumbar spondylosis.
• Bony malignant disease—in a man of this age, consider metastatic prostatic carcinoma and myeloma.
• Pelvic malignancy—metastatic carcinoma of the bladder or colon.
• Osteoporosis—although usually considered in women, older men are at risk, particularly if they have been treated with steroids. Pain from an osteoporotic fracture usually improves in about 3 weeks, but sequential vertebral crush fractures may present as chronic back pain.

History of the presenting problem

Oedema caused by heart failure

Specific symptoms of heart failure should be sought:
• Dyspnoea (this is less common in elderly people because their exercise tolerance is often limited)
• Orthopnoea (but older people may sleep propped up for reasons other than breathlessness)
• Paroxysmal nocturnal dyspnoea and nocturnal cough (can be confused with asthma or the major problem may be waking early with depression and then feeling breathless as usual)

• Fatigue and lethargy (common in heart failure but non-specific because it is common in many chronic diseases and cancer)

• Nausea and vomiting (may raise the suspicion of gastrointestinal pathology, but relatively common as a result of gastric congestion)

• Think about possible aetiology, remembering that there are often multiple predisposing and precipitating factors.

Causes of heart failure

• Coronary heart disease—prevalence increasing with better treatment of myocardial infarction.
• Hypertension.

Causes of heart failure (continued)

• Cardiomyopathy—dilated (alcohol), hypertrophic and restrictive (amyloidosis and haemochromatosis).
• Valve disease.
• Drugs—cardiac depressant drug, e.g. calcium antagonists and β-blockers.
• Dysrhythmias—both tachy- and bradydysrhythmias can precipitate heart failure.
• Right heart failure, e.g. recurrent pulmonary emboli and cor pulmonale.
• Pericardial disease.
• High-output states, e.g. anaemia, thyrotoxicosis and Paget's disease.
• Myocarditis—usually viral, e.g. Coxsackie, influenza.
(See *Cardiology*, Section 2.8.)

Case history example

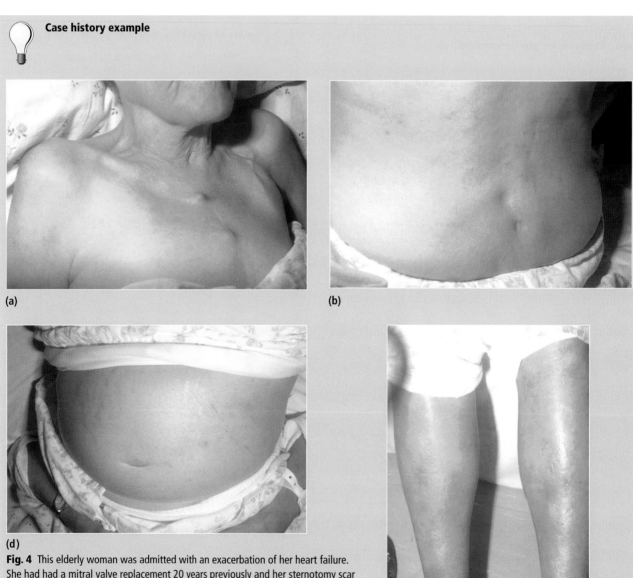

(a)

(b)

(d)

(c)

Fig. 4 This elderly woman was admitted with an exacerbation of her heart failure. She had had a mitral valve replacement 20 years previously and her sternotomy scar can be seen. She also has a permanent pacemaker which can be seen as a bulge in the left upper chest wall (a). Her jugular venous pressure was elevated and she had sacral (b) and peripheral (c) oedema and abdominal distension as the result of ascites. (d) The abdominal distension has resulted in striae that can be seen; the purple discoloration of her legs is varicose eczema caused by chronic venous insufficiency.

Specific questions may give clues. Sudden onset of breathlessness with the ankle swelling 6 weeks ago may have followed a painless infarct. Palpitations and a more gradual development of oedema may have followed the onset of atrial fibrillation. As with breathlessness, angina may not be a problem because of impaired mobility.

Causes of backache

Explore the possibilities:
- Ask about trauma/falls/fractures
- Prostatic cancer—urgency, nocturia, poor stream and terminal dribbling
- Myeloma—symptoms of hypercalcaemia, e.g. polyuria, polydipsia and constipation
- Bladder neoplasm—haematuria
- Colonic malignancy—altered bowel habit, abdominal pain, blood and mucus per rectum, and weight loss.

Relevant past history

Consider risk factors for ischaemic heart disease, particularly smoking, hypertension and diabetes. Other factors that are very significant in a young patient are less important in older people, e.g. family history and hyperlipidaemia. Is there other evidence of vascular disease such as transient ischaemic attacks or intermittent claudication? Elderly people still present with the sequelae of rheumatic heart disease so ask about childhood rheumatic fever, but most valve disease in this group now is the result of the effects of degenerative and ischaemic heart disease.

Social history

This man appears to have had little contact with any services and may be very isolated. Another explanation is that he has been fit and did not need help. It is important to establish how he was managing before admission and whether there are any immediate problems, e.g. whether he has pets to consider. Is alcohol a problem? Plan ahead for what he may need on discharge. Will he need time to regain independence in the activities of daily living (washing, dressing and food preparation)? Does he have a family who can help? Will he need social support, e.g. meals on wheels and home help? Is he eligible for extra income, e.g. attendance allowance? (see Section 2.12, p. 91).

Drug history

His medication may give some clues. What analgesia has he been using? This might tell you about the severity of the pain and complications may contribute to the clinical picture, e.g. NSAIDs may cause fluid retention, and renal impairment and chronic gastrointestinal blood loss may have led to severe anaemia. Has he been left on steroids after his 'bronchitis'? Remember to think about all routes of administration; β-blockers in eye drops can exacerbate cardiac failure and asthma.

Examination

General features

Look for the following:
- self-neglect—dementia or depression?
- undernutrition—common in heart failure and malignancy
- anaemia—pallor, angular stomatitis, glossitis
- malar flush—usually caused by exposure to the weather, but occasionally a sign of pulmonary hypertension, e.g. mitral stenosis
- tremor and palmar erythema—classically thyrotoxicosis, but consider alcohol
- jaundice—clinical jaundice is more likely to be the result of liver disease than congestion, although liver enzymes are often elevated in right heart failure
- xanthelasma—a sign of hyperlipidaemia, but most men with hyperlipidaemia do not survive to 79 years
- lymphadenopathy.

Cardiovascular assessment

A full assessment should be performed. The physical signs of heart failure are similar to those in younger patients. However, because of ageing changes and multiple pathology, signs may be difficult to interpret and interrater reliability for many signs is poor. The following are some useful points:
- Atrial fibrillation (AF) is common. In old age, the atrial contribution compensates for impaired diastolic filling, so loss of this with AF may precipitate heart failure.
- Signs of valve disease may be attenuated. The slow rising pulse and narrow pulse pressure of aortic stenosis may be affected by decreased arterial compliance.
- The altered shape of the chest wall in kyphosis and chronic lung disease alters the classic radiation of murmurs and the position of the apex beat.
- Basal crackles in the chest are non-specific.

Abdomen

Hepatomegaly and ascites may be present in severe heart failure. These signs may also be the result of malignancy. You should look for masses in the abdomen and genitalia, and for lymph nodes in the groins if the oedema is thought to be caused by lymphatic obstruction, and perform a rectal examination to check the size and consistency of the prostate and for a rectal mass.

Other aspects

Examine the legs and sacrum if the swelling extends above the thighs or the patient has been in bed. Lymphoedema is usually distinguishable from pitting oedema but chronic 'pitting' oedema pits less well! Cellulitis and DVT may have caused the swelling or be a complication of cardiac failure. Where is the back pain? Examine the spine and look for neurological signs in the legs.

- Gross leg oedema may be missed if previous recurrent cellulitis has made the ankles so 'woody' that the skin cannot expand. Look further up the leg.
- If one leg is more swollen than the other, check for DVT or previous history, the scar of hip surgery or a stroke affecting that side or a tremor, e.g. Parkinson's disease, affecting the 'thin' leg.

Approach to investigations and management

Investigations

All patients with heart failure need an FBC, electrolytes and renal function, liver function, glucose and thyroid function tests. Check cardiac enzymes if a recent myocardial infarction is suspected. It is uncertain whether it is worth measuring lipids at his age; there is no evidence for the efficacy of treatment, but this is not the same as evidence of no benefit.

A chest radiograph, ECG and echocardiogram are indicated and 24-hour Holter monitoring is useful if intermittent arrhythmias are suspected. Figures 5 and 6 show typical chest radiographic findings in cardiac failure. The ECG is abnormal in 90% of cases. Common abnormalities are: Q waves, T and ST segment changes, left ventricular hypertrophy, bundle-branch block and atrial fibrillation. ST elevation may indicate recent infarction but, if it is persistent, it is a sign of a left ventricular aneurysm which can also be complicated by

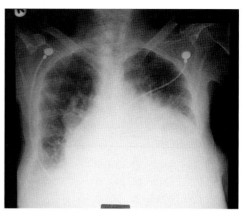

Fig. 5 Chest radiograph showing gross cardiomegaly and pulmonary oedema.

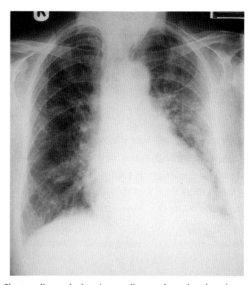

Fig. 6 Chest radiograph showing cardiomegaly and early pulmonary oedema with upper lobe diversion and increased lung markings of interalveolar oedema (Kerley B lines).

heart failure (Fig. 7). The echocardiogram is a useful non-invasive test to detect and assess valvular disease and left ventricular function. Rare causes of heart failure may be detected, e.g. atrial myxoma (Figs 8 and 9).

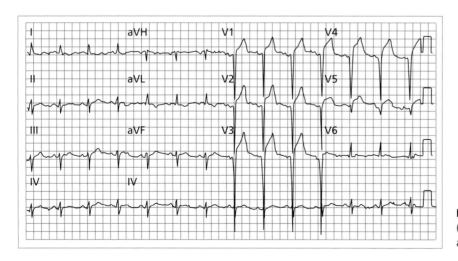

Fig. 7 ECG showing anteroseptal ST elevation (leads V1–V5). This patient had a left ventricular aneurysm.

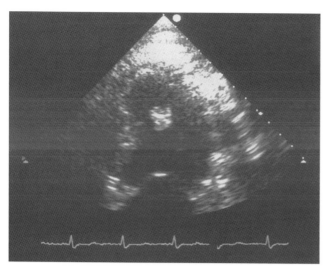

Fig. 8 Two-dimensional echocardiogram showing the left ventricle which is aneurysmal at its apex. The high density around the lesion in the apex is a thrombus in the aneurysm.

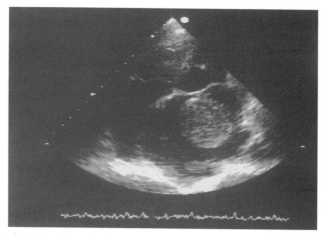

Fig. 9 Two-dimensional echocardiogram: parasternal long axis view. The round 'tennis ball'-like density in the left atrium is an atrial myxoma.

In this patient, the leg swelling was part of the picture of chronic heart failure but this would not explain the back pain, unless he had fallen because of his heavy legs. Tests should be sent for prostate cancer and myeloma (see Section 1.5, p. 62) and other investigations arranged as indicated by the findings. A Doppler scan of the leg veins is needed to exclude major DVT. In this patient, the prostate was craggy and the prostate-specific antigen (PSA) was high. Lumbar spine films were equivocal but a bone scan showed multiple secondaries, particularly in the spine and left hip.

Management

The overall management plan will include management of the heart failure (see below) and prostate cancer. Involve the urologists and cancer services. Treatment will probably include a gonadorelin analogue, with initial antiandrogen cover to prevent flare, pain control and radiotherapy. Although he is acutely ill, remember prevention: avoid pressure sores, give subcutaneous heparin and arrange nutritional supplements. He will need input from the multidisciplinary team and a period of rehabilitation before careful discharge planning.

 He is likely to die from his heart failure before his prostate cancer; good symptom control is often lacking in terminal heart and lung disease.

Management of heart failure

Management is similar to that in younger patients (see *Cardiology*, Section 2.8), but with a different emphasis. Lifestyle changes and drugs for secondary prevention are only worthwhile if the patient has a reasonable prognosis. Encourage patients with cardiac cachexia to eat whatever they fancy and graze! Exercise programmes may be particularly valuable in elderly people in whom lack of fitness may make a major contribution to their symptoms.

DRUG MANAGEMENT

 The proportion of patients with heart failure caused by diastolic dysfunction (stiff ventricle) is not known, although it is more common in old age. There are no data to guide specific management.

Diuretics
Thiazide or loop diuretics are usually used as the first line of treatment to control symptoms, but they have never been shown to reduce mortality. Intravenous treatment will be needed if there is gastric congestion. Watch the potassium, especially if the patient is on digoxin. In severe resistant oedema, the combination of metolazone and a loop diuretic may be very effective but start with 2.5 mg metolazone, because the diuresis may be drastic. Reduce the diuretics before the patient reaches his 'dry weight' or you will overshoot. When the patient is stable, metolazone may be useful intermittently, e.g. twice a week.

 Your patient has lost 10 kg in weight, his ankles are slim, his blood pressure acceptable, and his electrolytes and renal function satisfactory. You are delighted but he insists that he still feels awful. Don't despair and encourage him. Patients often take about a week to feel better!

Angiotensin-converting enzyme inhibitors
All patients with left ventricular systolic dysfunction should receive these drugs unless there is a contraindication

because many studies have shown that they reduce morbidity, mortality and hospital admissions.

 When adding an ACE inhibitor, proceed with caution. Aortic and renal artery stenosis are more common in old age. Check that patient is not dry, give a trial dose, often captopril 6.25 mg in the evening, and watch for hypotension and renal impairment. A dose that is well tolerated when the patient is stable may cause renal failure if another problem such as a chest infection supervenes. However, if the ACE inhibitor is well tolerated, increase the dose to the therapeutic range.

Nitrates and hydralazine

If the patient is intolerant of ACE inhibitors, this combination should be considered because it has been shown to reduce mortality.

Digoxin

This is the drug of choice to control the rate in established atrial fibrillation and has also been shown to be inotropic in the presence of sinus rhythm. It reduces hospital admissions in those with heart failure, but has not been shown to have an effect on mortality.

Spironolactone

Provided that there are no contraindications, the addition of spironolactone to treatment with diuretics, ACE inhibitors and digoxin has been shown to reduce mortality in moderate-to-severe heart failure.

Beta-blockers

In recent trials, these drugs have been shown to reduce morbidity and mortality. They should be used with care by a specialist and may be contraindicated in many elderly smokers because of chronic obstructive pulmonary disease (COPD) and peripheral vascular disease.

 Heart failure drugs: what's new? *Drug Ther Bull* 2000; 38: 25–27. This review gives the primary sources for the range of treatments listed above.

1.7 Gradual decline

Case history

The daughter of an 85-year-old retired telephonist is concerned about her mother who has been living with her for 2 years. She just sits in her chair, appears apathetic and naps throughout the day. She is intermittently confused.

Clinical approach

These symptoms are non-specific and could be the result of a wide range of conditions. The causes of drowsiness and apathy overlap with those of acute and chronic confusion (see Sections 1.2, p. 53 and 2.7, p. 83).

 Causes of drowsiness / tiredness

- Drugs, e.g. 'hangover' effect of sedatives, antidepressants and neuroleptics, and side effects of other drugs, e.g. anticonvulsants, codeine, etc.
- Alcohol.
- Psychiatric problems, particularly depression and dementia.
- Infections, e.g. urinary tract, after pneumonia or influenza.
- Chronic disease especially with an acute phase response, e.g. malignancy and rheumatoid disease.
- Metabolic and endocrine problems, e.g. hypothyroidism, diabetes mellitus, hyponatraemia.
- Intracranial pathology (especially lesions causing a pressure effect, e.g. frontal tumour, subdural haematoma, rarely tuberculous meningitis, abscess).
- Chronic organ failure, e.g. respiratory failure, renal failure and cardiac failure, may present insidiously.
- Severe anaemia.

History of the presenting problem

A fuller history from the daughter is essential. How long has her mother been deteriorating and were there any precipitating factors? When did her husband die and what is her mood like? She is described as intermittently confused, but does she appear to have dementia? The situation has been worsening for 10 months, she has gained weight and is reluctant to get out of her chair. Her only medication is iron tablets. This information makes some of the options (drugs, infection, malignancy and chronic inflammatory disease) less likely. The final straw from the daughter's perspective is faecal soiling and she now feels that a nursing home is the only option. The patient herself has nothing to add to the history but doesn't think that anything is the matter.

Relevant past history

The daughter is vague, but the GP letter has a crucial fact—years ago she had a partial thyroidectomy.

Examination

The diagnosis that would explain all the features is hypothyroidism and you examine her with this in mind. You need to evaluate her mood and cognition (depression and dementia are both exacerbated by hypothyroidism). However, she may have other significant pathology that has been overlooked because of her general decline, so she needs a thorough examination. In particular, examine her abdomen and rectum (she has a distended bladder and faecal impaction) and her neurology. Here, the faecal soiling was the result of overflow, but may also occur when confused patients attempt manual disimpaction themselves.

 A clinical diagnosis of hypothyroidism is unreliable in elderly people, so always check thyroid function. However, some of the more useful signs are:
- alopecia (Fig. 10)
- dry, non-pitting thickened skin (infiltration of mucopolysaccharides)
- erythema ab igne—as she 'feels the cold', the patient has sat near to a fire for months (Fig. 11)
- slow relaxation of ankle jerks
- bilateral carpal tunnel syndrome
- signs of associated autoimmune disease, e.g. vitiligo (Fig. 12)
- signs of previous thyrotoxicosis, e.g. thyroidectomy scar, eye signs.

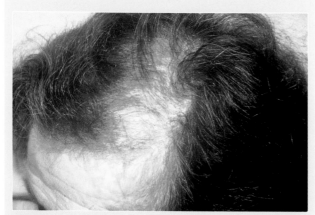

Fig. 10 Diffuse alopecia.

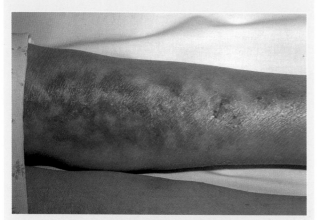

Fig. 11 Erythema ab igne: excoriation can be seen in this lesion which needs to be monitored because malignancy occasionally occurs.

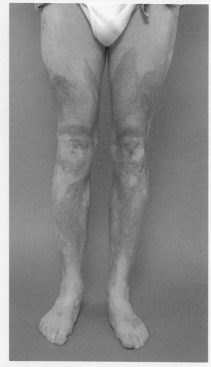

Fig. 12 Vitiligo.

Approach to investigations and management

Investigations

Blood tests include thyroid function tests (TSH is elevated and thyroxine low), FBC (anaemia may be normocytic or macrocytic but never megaloblastic, so check vitamin B_{12} if this is a finding), urea and electrolytes (dehydration may be present because of poor oral intake) and glucose. A partial thyroidectomy was probably performed for a nodule but check thyroid autoantibodies if relevant. The chest radiograph may show pleural or pericardial effusions. The ECG may show low-voltage complexes and sinus bradycardia. There may be flattening or inverted T waves. If there is associated hypothermia, look for a J wave.

Management

This situation has taken a long time to develop and a month of treatment may be needed before there is much evidence of benefit. It may be possible to keep the patient at home with home nursing and therapy, but admission to a slow stream rehabilitation unit may be the best option. However, ensure that the daughter expects her mother to improve and return home eventually. Begin replacement therapy with thyroxine 25 µg once a day, increasing by 25 µg increments every 14 days. The usual maintenance dose is 100–150 µg daily.

More rapid increases in thyroxine can cause tachydysrhythmias and precipitate a myocardial infarction or heart failure.

The faecal impaction will need treatment with enemas and then large doses of laxatives (softeners and stimulants) for a long period. Poor diet, dehydration and immobility will have compounded the effect of the hypothyroidism. Until the thyroxine begins to take effect, care will be needed to make sure that she does not deteriorate further and the full multidisciplinary team should be involved in her rehabilitation and safe discharge home.

 Chiovato L, Mariotti S, Pinchera A. Thyroid diseases in the elderly. *Baillière's Clin Endocrinol Metab* 1997; 11: 251–270.
Wallace K, Hofmann MT. Thyroid dysfunction: how to manage overt and subclinical disease in older patients. *Geriatrics* 1998; 53: 32–38.

2 Diseases and treatments

2.1 Why elderly patients are different

Many diseases in elderly people are a continuum of diseases found in middle age, so why are elderly patients different? How old is old? It depends on your perspective and where you live. Expectations of health and lifestyle are changing. In the UK now, most frail elderly people are aged over 80 [1]. Younger patients who are 'biologically old' with multisystem pathology often have arteriopathy or are 'graduates' with chronic disability.

 It is not how old you are, but how you are old. (Marie Dressler)

The effects of pathology are superimposed on the ageing process and influenced by fitness and social factors. Ageing changes are seen in most organs (Fig. 13).

Why do ageing changes matter?

In comparison with a group of younger people, in old age there is:
- increased variability between individuals
- impaired homeostasis: OK at rest, significant when stressed (e.g. fasting glucose minimally higher in elderly people, but glucose levels much higher after meals)
- different significance of some physical signs.

 After a post-take ward round, reflect on the different individuals you have seen of similar chronological age.

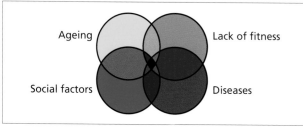

Fig. 13 The background of disease in old age.

Multiple pathology

In young adults, you try to fit all the symptoms and signs to one condition. The situation is different in elderly people [2], a fact recognized since antiquity.

 How incessant and great are the ills with which a prolonged old age is replete. (Juvenal)

Why do old people often have several diseases?

The prevalence of many diseases increases with age, e.g. stroke and Alzheimer's disease. There is more time for things to accrue so this may be chance, but not all occurrences will be random. Disparate conditions may have a common pathogenesis, e.g. failure to mop up free radicals, which could be influenced genetically (isoenzyme activities) or environmentally (dietary antioxidant). A given genotype may be associated with several conditions. Commonly occurring risk factors (e.g. smoking) predispose to several diseases. Some chronic diseases have complications affecting several systems (e.g. diabetes) or predispose to other things (e.g. infection).

Different risk factors

A risk factor in middle-aged individuals may not carry the same risk in old age. Data from trials of antihypertensives including progressively older cohorts have established hypertension as a vascular risk factor up to around 80 years of age. HYVET, the HYpertension in the Very Elderly Trial, co-ordinated by Chris Bulpitt, is currently recruiting subjects aged over 80 [3]. The situation with high cholesterol remains unclear.

Different susceptibility to disease

Tuberculosis is more common in elderly people (reasons may include socioeconomic factors, prior exposure, changes in the immune system, etc.). Nosocomial *Clostridium difficile* diarrhoea is more common in frail elderly than in middle-aged people, so departments of medicine and of medicine for elderly people often have different antibiotic policies.

 Find out about antibiotic policies in medicine and medicine for elderly people in your hospital.

Table 3 Likely causes of fits and jaundice in different age groups.

	Likely cause	
	Fits	Jaundice
Neonate	Birth trauma, hypoxia	Physiological
Baby/toddler	Fever	Biliary atresia
Child/teenager	Epilepsy	Hepatitis A
Young adult	Drugs, alcohol or withdrawal	Drugs, alcohol
Middle age	Brain tumour	Gallstones
Old age	Cerebrovascular disease	Carcinoma of the pancreas

Different differential diagnoses

Listing the diagnostic possibilities in the probable order for a particular individual is a challenge for newly qualified doctors and for more experienced doctors in the heat of an examination. Ethnic background is important—worldwide, the most common cause of iron deficiency anaemia is hookworm, but this is rare in East Anglia! Age is another major factor to consider before reeling off your list of probabilities (Table 3).

Altered response to disease

Illness in old age may have a typical presentation, but not always—an intellectual challenge of the specialty. Most of the public can diagnose serious pathology in middle age (e.g. when the postman collapsed, nearby builders recognized his symptoms and dialled 999). However, spotting a heart attack or pneumonia in elderly people can be more tricky:

• Missing symptoms, e.g. pain may be absent in a myocardial infarction, perforated viscus (air under the diaphragm on a chest radiograph is a surprise finding) and attenuation of thirst, predisposing to dehydration.
• Missing signs, e.g. fever may be absent despite serious infection, neck stiffness absent in purulent meningitis.
• Non-specific or atypical presentation, e.g. confusion, is common.

Non-specific presentation of disease

The following could all be presentations of an acute problem (e.g. stroke), a chronic condition (e.g. Parkinson's disease) or a new analgesic:

• instability (falls)
• incontinence
• intellectual failure (confusion)
• immobility—'off her feet'
• failure to thrive.

The 'geriatric giants' or five 'I's are:
• intellectual failure
• incontinence
• immobility
• instability
• iatrogenic disease.

The presenting condition is often complicated by the consequences of immobility, particularly after a long lie (e.g. incontinence, dehydration, pressure sores, DVT, risk of compartment syndrome, rhabdomyolysis).

Inappropriate prescribing and polypharmacy

Contraindications to a drug, side effects, adverse events and drug interactions are all more common in old age (see Section 2.6, p. 82).

Social problems

There are sadder aspects. Old age is a time of loss, not necessarily balanced by the compensations of a fulfilling life and supportive family. Retirement is a recent phenomenon. This 'luxury' of a civilized society can leave an individual without a role, with reduced income and status, and a falling standard of living, with enforced membership of a group described as a 'rising tide', a 'burden' or even an 'epidemic'. Western culture now values youth and beauty above wisdom and experience. Listen, share and focus on the practical problems that result and how they affect the patient. What might help? Don't make assumptions, particularly in different ethnic groups.

Expectations

Things are changing (some parts of the USA are way ahead), but elderly patients may have low expectations for their health and of the system. Problems such as swollen ankles or incontinence are attributed to 'old age'. Elderly patients are not infrequently admitted with anasarca. Ankle swelling spreads to the thighs and trunk before help is sought. It takes time to shift the fluid, but patients can often be discharged on small doses of loop diuretic and an ACE inhibitor. The cardiac failure was not severe, just neglected. Families may have low expectations but some expect miracles. Professionals in all disciplines may have ageist attitudes: 'well, my dear, what do you expect at your age?' Where resources are short, the old are frequently at the end of the queue. Ageism should be as unacceptable as racism, but common-sense **is** required.

Age Concern website: www.ace.org.uk
Help the Aged website: www.helptheaged.org.uk
Centre for Policy on Ageing website: www.cpa.org.uk
National Institute of Aging (USA) website: www.nih.gov/nia
1 Evans JG, Williams TF, eds. *Oxford Textbook of Geriatric Medicine*, 2nd edn. Oxford: Oxford University Press, 2000. A standard reference textbook.
2 Palmer RM. Geriatric assessment. *Med Clin North Am* 1999; 83: 1503–1523.
3 Bulpitt CJ, Fletcher AE, Amery A *et al*. The Hypertension in the Very Elderly Trial (HYVET). Rationale, methodology and comparison with previous trials. *Lancet* 1999; 353: 793–796.

2.2 General approach to management

History

Obtaining an accurate history may require detective work and the history needs to extend beyond the presenting problem:
• Several informants, e.g. phone the home help/GP
• Social history, especially what could she do before she was ill?
• Medication (prescribed and OTC).

Examination

In many other specialties the examination, especially when done by a consultant in outpatients, is very focused, but in a frail older patient:
• Examination is usually comprehensive rather than targeted to one system
• Rushing is counterproductive
• Beware of short cuts—take the socks off, look under bandages
• Remember the rectal examination
• Assess cognition, function and mood.

Investigations

Remember why you are doing investigations, i.e. to confirm diagnoses, look for complications and as a baseline for therapy. In a stressful situation (examinations) or when you feel overwhelmed (you have identified seven different problems), it helps to think of tests in groups and work from the basic to the complex.

Most geriatricians use a mix of specific and 'screening' tests when a patient is admitted to hospital because of the prevalence of non-specific presentation and unexpected pathology:

• Urine tests
• Blood tests (think by laboratory—haematology, biochemistry, etc.)
• Other specimens for bacteriology
• Chest radiograph
• ECG
• Other tests, e.g. echocardiography, 24-hour tape, tilt testing, lung function, endoscopy, EEG, EMG
• Imaging—plain radiographs, ultrasonography, contrast studies, CT, MRI, positron emission tomography (PET), etc.
• Histology? With the expansion in imaging, tissue diagnosis may be delayed.

Once the results of the basic investigations are available it is important to take stock.

• What am I dealing with?
• What is treatable?
• What is important? (to the patient and carer as well as to the doctor)
• Don't lose sight of the wood for the trees!

Management

Summarize the situation and decide on a plan of action. Management almost always involves the multidisciplinary team and the process of rehabilitation to maximize the function (physical, mental and social) of the individual patient (see Section 2.8, p. 85).

Consider the following:
• Education (patients' societies can be very useful)
• Physiotherapy, speech and language therapy, occupational therapy, dietitian, podiatry (chiropody)
• Social services
• Improve general health (remember eyes and ears, nutrition)
• Treat other treatable conditions
• Specific drug treatment
• Control of remaining symptoms
• Support for the carer.

End of life decisions

For these, see the BMA guidelines [1]. Each decision about when to move from cure to care is unique, but there are some general principles. It may be hard for doctors to accept the inevitable, particularly if there is no clear diagnosis (easier in cancer) and if earlier management was suboptimal.

In the name of Hippocrates, doctors have invented the most exquisite form of torture ever known to man: survival.
(Luis Buñuel)

The decision should not be placed on the family, and legally remains the responsibility of the consultant, but it would be foolish to ignore the views of the multidisciplinary team. Good communication with the patient, family and team is essential. Do not take away hope, but reassure that symptom control is paramount (see Section 1.4, p. 60 and *Palliative care*, Sections 2.9 and 2.10).

Do Not Resuscitate orders

The decision not to perform cardiopulmonary resuscitation is not the same as the decision to withhold active treatment, but the two are sometimes confused. Many patients who would not be resuscitated in the event of a cardiorespiratory arrest receive a whole range of other treatments.

It has been recommended that all DNR decisions should be discussed with the patient and the family. However, this discussion is not an easy one. On admission, elderly patients who are ill, but not expecting to die, may be distressed by the concept, however well handled. Later in their stay, patients may interpret this discussion as evidence that things are much worse than you have let on. The family view is important, but relatives may not be available and may disagree among themselves, and your primary duty is to the patient. Doctors are not obliged to discuss futile treatments with patients and the results of resuscitation in non-cardiac care unit (CCU) settings are poor. Chronological age itself is not a reason for a DNR decision. However, the burden of pathology in many elderly patients often makes resuscitation inappropriate because the patient is so unlikely to survive the procedure or a stay in an intensive therapy unit and return home. As a junior, find out your consultant's policy, be aware of your hospital guidelines and always discuss a DNR decision with the nursing staff. If death is likely, plan to talk things over with the family (suggested timing is discussed in Section 1.4, p. 60).

Communication with colleagues. Try to plan ahead and record decisions clearly in the notes so that covering teams know the plan if your patient deteriorates. Different levels of intervention may be appropriate, e.g. 'for intravenous antibiotics, but not for a central line or ventilation'.

1 British Medical Association. *Withholding and Withdrawing Life-prolonging Medical Treatment: Guidance for Decision Making*. London: BMJ Books, 1999.

2.3 Falls

Falls are:
- very common
- significant causes of morbidity and mortality
- often preventable
- a marker of failing function.

Epidemiology

Almost a third of those aged over 65 years have at least one fall per year:
- The incidence increases with age so that 50% of those aged over 85 years fall every year
- Women fall more often than men
- Falls may be a marker of acute illness: myocardial infarct, pulmonary embolus, pneumonia or a urinary tract infection
- Falls may be a sign of chronic illness, including anaemia, myxoedema and dementia.

Aetiology

Falls are usually multifactorial, so all contributing factors need to be identified [1]. People with dementia are at particular risk of falls, but remediable causes must still be sought, especially side effects of psychotropic medication (Table 4).

Clinical presentation

The history may point to the systems involved:
- Examine the relevant systems
- Always check vision, hearing, gait, feet and shoes, and postural blood pressure
- Check for any injuries
- Drugs: hepatic drug extraction and metabolism, and most significantly glomerular filtration rate, all slow with age, so elderly people are more susceptible to adverse effects.

Being on four or more different medications correlates most strongly with a high risk of falling (Table 5).

Investigations

General investigations depend on what was found in the history and examination.

Tilt-table testing may be useful in sorting out the causes of syncope. Measurement of beat-to-beat variation in pulse and BP may indicate carotid hypersensitivity or a vasodepressor response [2].

Table 4 Causes, investigation and management of falls.

System	Associated symptoms	Signs	Investigations	Causes	Treatments
Cardiovascular	Transient loss of consciousness, with rapid recovery, but may have retrograde amnesia	Slow pulse	ECG Holter monitor	Bradyarrhythmia/ complete heart block	Permanent pacing
	Palpitations	Fast atrial fibrillation	ECG Holter monitor	Symptomatic tachyarrhythmia, e.g. paroxysmal atrial fibrillation	Anti-arrhythmic therapy
	None/angina/breathlessness	Ejection systolic murmur	Echocardiogram	Aortic stenosis	Aortic valve replacement
	Dizziness on standing	Drop of >20 mmHg systolic or >10 diastolic BP after standing for 2 min	Consider: tilt table Synacthen test	Postural hypotension: secondary to drugs, Addison's disease, autonomic neuropathy, e.g. diabetes	Stop diuretics and anti-hypertensives, try TED stockings, fludrocortisone
	Acute nausea, vomiting followed by a transient loss of consciousness with rapid recovery	Pale and clammy		Vasovagal episode	
Neurological	Unilateral weakness	Hemiplegia, carotid bruit	CT brain scan	Stroke	Secondary prevention
	Loss of consciousness with incontinence, tongue biting and postictal drowsiness or confusion	Tonic–clonic movements bilateral upgoing plantars	EEG CT brain scan	Epilepsy	Antiepileptic therapy
	Difficulty turning over in bed, tremor, poverty of movement, drooling	Mask-like facies, pill-rolling tremor, cogwheel rigidity, flexed posture, festinant gait	CT brain scan to exclude atherosclerotic pseudo-parkinsonism	Idiopathic Parkinson's disease	Levodopa therapy, dopamine agonists, COMT inhibitors
	Confusion, incontinence	Broad-based gait	CT brain scan	Normal pressure hydrocephalus	VP shunt
	Difficulty getting out of a chair	Weakness of proximal muscles	TSH	Proximal myopathy	Thyroid disease

Table 4 continued.

System	Associated symptoms	Signs	Investigations	Causes	Treatments
Psychiatric diseases	Low mood	Flat affect	Geriatric Depression Scale	Depression	Antidepressants
	Poor memory, confusion	May be signs of previous strokes	CT brain scan TSH, vitamin B_{12}, folate	Vascular dementia, Alzheimer's disease, Lewy body dementia	Review medication
Decreased sensory input and balance disturbance	Poor vision	Visual acuity fields Fundoscopy	Ophthalmology review	Presbyopia, glaucoma, macular degeneration, cataracts, diabetic retinopathy	Spectacles of correct prescription Treatment for glaucoma Cataract extraction Laser therapy if indicated
	Deafness	Wax in canal, perforated drum	Audiometry, CT brain scan	Presbycousis, wax, otosclerosis, acoustic neuroma	Remove wax Hearing aid (check batteries)
	Dizziness	BP, waxy ears, anaemia	FBC, CT brain scan	Drugs, CVA	Stop drugs, treat cause
	Vertigo	Positive Hallpike manoeuvre		BPPV	Vestibular rehabilitation

BP, blood pressure; BPPV, benign paroxysmal positional vertigo; COMT, catecholamine-*O*-methyltransferase; CT, computed tomographic; CVA, cerebrovascular accident; EEG, electroencephalography; FBC, full blood count; TED, thromboembolic device; TSH, thyroid-stimulating hormone; VP, ventriculoperitoneal shunt.

Table 5 Drugs associated with increased risk of falling.

Class	Effect	Example	Possible solution
Antipsychotic medication	Sedation	Chlorpromazine	Try atypical such as risperidone
	Extrapyramidal effects	Haloperidol	
	Postural hypotension	Chlorpromazine	Avoid co-prescribing with diuretics
Tricyclic antidepressants	Postural hypotension	Lofepramine, amitriptyline	SSRIs are less likely to cause dysrhythmias
	Arrhythmias		and *may* cause less hypotension
Analgesics	Sedation	Opiates	Try non-opiate, e.g. paracetamol, given regularly
Antiepileptic drugs	Overdosage causes cerebellar side effects	Phenytoin, carbamazepine	Monitor levels
Alcohol	Acute intoxication causes reduced level of consciousness		Education
	Chronic abuse causes cerebellar damage		Thiamine therapy
	Acute withdrawal causes acute confusion		High index of suspicion, protect with reducing doses of chlordiazepoxide on admission
Benzodiazepines	Sedation. Acute withdrawal can cause confusion and falls	Diazepam, nitrazepam	Avoid if possible. If withdrawal symptoms suspected, slowly reduce the dose
Cardiovascular medications	Low BP	Diuretics, nitrates, other vasodilators	Use lowest therapeutic dose
Parkinson's disease medication	Postural hypotension	Levodopa preparations: Madopar, Sinemet Dopamine agonists: pergolide	Co-prescribe fludrocortisone, TED stockings

BP, blood pressure; SSRI, selective serotonin reuptake inhibitor; TED, thromboembolic device.

Treatment

 The best strategy for preventing falls is by multiple interventions [3,4].

Review all medications. Are they necessary? Are they causing interactions? Are they causing postural hypotension? Treat all contributing factors.

Refer to an occupational therapist, who will:
• assess the patient's home for accessibility, adequate lighting, and advise on the removal of potential hazards (e.g. mats on shiny floors, loose wires, clutter, pets)
• arrange for the provision of appropriate aids such as a toilet raise, trolley for transporting drinks and food from room to room, perching stools for tasks such as washing, cooking, etc.
• assess the patient's ability to look after herself.

Refer to the physiotherapist, who will advise on whether walking aids will help the patient mobilize more safely, teach people how to get up once they have fallen and encourage balance training exercises such as Tai Chi.

The social worker will arrange a package of care to meet the needs of the individual.

Complications

Falls result in significant morbidity and mortality. Complications include the following:
• Decreased mobility, leading to potential for pressure sores, DVTs, incontinence and even contractures in severe cases
• Minor injury in 20% of those who fall
• Loss of confidence may deter people from leaving their homes (or concerned relatives may encourage them not to); this can be addressed by encouraging exercise and attendance at a day centre
• Low mood
• Decreased quality of life
• A significant proportion of elderly people who present to A&E after a fall are admitted
• Five per cent sustain a fracture; therefore, consider prevention of osteoporosis with calcium and vitamin D or bisphosphonates, or the use of hip protector pads [5]
• Recurrent falls may eventually lead to people being institutionalized prematurely.

Information for patients

Refer patients to suitable sources of information [6,7].

1 Tinetti ME, Speechley M, Ginter SF. Risk factors for falls among elderly people in the community. *N Engl J Med* 1988; 319: 1701–1709.
2 Parry SW, Kenny RA. Tilt table testing in the diagnosis of unexplained syncope. *Q J Med* 1999; 92: 623–629.
3 Tinetti ME, Baker DI, Mcavey G *et al.* A multifactorial intervention to reduce the risk of falling among elderly people living in the community. *N Engl J Med* 1994; 331: 821–827.
4 Close J, Ellis E, Hooper R, Glucksman E, Jackson S, Swift C. Prevention of Falls in the Elderly Trial (PROFET). *Lancet* 1999; 353: 93–97.
5 Wilkinson TJ, Sainsbury R. Hip protectors. *Age Ageing* 1998; 27: 89–90.
6 *Falls: How to Avoid Them and How to Cope.* Royal Society for the Prevention of Accidents and Age Concern.
7 *Growing Older Safely.* Royal Society for the Prevention of Accidents.

2.4 Urinary and faecal incontinence

2.4.1 URINARY INCONTINENCE

Urinary incontinence is defined as 'the involuntary loss of urine sufficient in volume or frequency to be a social or a health problem'.

Urinary incontinence is:
- very common
- often concealed by the patient
- a major cause of poor quality of life
- an important factor contributing to institutionalization
- an enormous burden both to the individual and to society
- often treatable.

Aetiology and pathophysiology

Table 6 lists the causes and management of different types of incontinence. Several factors make urinary incontinence more likely.

Table 6 Causes and management of different types of incontinence.

Type	Symptoms	Examination findings	Investigations	Causes	Treatments
Stress incontinence	Involuntary leaking of small amounts of urine on coughing, laughing, exercising	Vaginal examination: cystocele, vaginal prolapse	MSU, stable bladder on cystoscopy, leakage on stress testing	Multiparity, pelvic surgery in women, prostate surgery in men, collagen disorders	Exercises to strengthen pelvic floor. Ring pessaries. Surgical procedures
Urge incontinence	Overwhelming and instant urge to pass urine with involuntary emptying of the bladder	No specific findings	MSU, unstable detrusor contractions during cystometry	Detrusor instability caused by ageing, or hyperreflexia in neurological disease, e.g. MS, CVA, PD	Anticholinergic drugs: tolterodine, oxybutynin, imipramine. Desmopressin
Mixed	Symptoms of both stress and urge incontinence	Signs as above	Mixture of above	Mixture of above	Treat for urge incontinence first, then stress
Overflow incontinence	Constant dribbling, sensation that the bladder is not empty	Palpable bladder, faecal loading in either sex, enlarged prostate in men, cystocele in women	Enlarged bladder with large residual volume	Prostatism, urethral, stricture, bladder overdistension, faecal loading. Drugs	Surgical relief of the obstruction (e.g. TURP, urethral dilatation). Cholinomimetics such as bethanecol. Catheters
Functional and iatrogenic	Inability to reach the toilet secondary to reduced mobility, confusion	Signs of underlying disease	Normal ultrasonography and urodynamics	Arthritis, PD, CVA, acute confusion, dementia, plaster cast, drugs, etc.	Treat underlying problem. Change drugs. Commode, toilet raise, pad and pants, conveen, catheter

MS, multiple sclerosis; MSU, midstream urine sample; TURP, transurethral prostatectomy; PD, Parkinson's disease; CVA, cerebrovascular accident.

General age-related changes

- Reduced bladder capacity.
- Increase in residual volume.
- Increased number of bladder spasms (detrusor contractions).
- Change in the normal diurnal production of anti-diuretic hormone, so that less is produced at night, leading to nocturia.
- Decreased mobility.

Sex-related changes

Being female increases the risk of incontinence for several reasons:

- Anatomy—the longer urethra and presence of the prostate gland enhance continence in men; the short urethra in women increases the risk of UTI
- Multiparity—vaginal delivery of large babies, with stretching and perineal tears and inadequate pelvic floor exercises afterwards, leads to weakness of the pelvic floor and hypermobility of the neck of the bladder
- Postmenopausally—the fall in oestrogen leads to reduced smooth muscle tone in the urethra, a higher pH permits pathogens to flourish and dryness causes the sensation of urgency, as well as dyspareunia
- Concurrent drug treatments (see Table 2, p. 32)
- Acute and chronic confusional states
- Co-morbid diseases, e.g. diabetes.

Epidemiology

Urinary incontinence is very common and not just confined to elderly people. It can affect the following:

- 10% of the general population
- 20% of those aged over 70 years (probably an underestimate)
- twice as common in women
- very common in people living in nursing homes
- only 25% of affected women consult a doctor [1].

Clinical presentation

See Section 1.3, p. 56.

Investigations

If incontinence persists despite simple measures, further investigation is indicated:

- Urodynamic investigation—measures free flow rate and residual volume.
- Cystometry—the bladder is filled at a steady rate while recording the difference between the intra-abdominal and intravesical pressures; this is the detrusor pressure,

which will be increased if there are uninhibited detrusor contractions, leading to urgency.
- Cystoscopy will reveal causes of bladder irritation and haematuria, such as bladder stones, interstitial cystitis and transitional cell carcinoma.

 It is important to establish the cause of the incontinence. Although general measures, e.g. treat constipation, are the same, the exercise regimens and the drug management depend on the type of incontinence. Drugs for the treatment of urge incontinence are contraindicated in prostatic outflow obstruction.

Treatment

General principles that should be applied to most patients:
- Regular toileting, initially voiding every 1–1.5 hours
- Bladder retraining: the patient gradually increases the time between voiding
- Limit fluid intake to 1.5 L per day
- Oestrogen replacement for symptoms of atrophic vaginitis, used topically for local problems but orally for general symptoms of oestrogen deficiency
- Avoid bladder irritants, e.g. caffeine, alcohol and aspartame
- Improve the patient's mobility where possible
- Increase the accessibility of toilets: toilet raise, rails, wide doors, large sign on the door and Continence Society cards (easy access to the facilities in town)
- Consider a commode: urine bottle for men, various designs of slipper pans for women
- Choose sensible clothes, e.g. Velcro fastenings.

Stress incontinence

Non-surgical

- Exercises, e.g. Kegel's exercises (concentrate on contracting the pelvic floor to interrupt the flow of urine), do work, but they require the patient to be cognitively intact and motivated.
- Vaginal cones (weights placed in the vagina to help with targeting pelvic floor exercises), biofeedback (detrusor spasms are converted to a signal that the patient can see or hear and tries to suppress) and electrical stimulation of the pudendal nerve have been shown not to improve continence significantly.

Surgical

- Periurethral collagen injections—can be done using local anaesthetic and oral sedation.
- Repositioning of the bladder neck—anterior repair or colposuspension, usually under general anaesthetic.
- Endoscopic needle suspension of the bladder neck—less invasive, but the long-term cure rate is low.

Urge incontinence

Several groups of drugs may be tried but this should always be in addition to the general measures:
• Oxybutinin and tolterodine are the drugs most often prescribed. They are anticholinergic (antimuscarinic) and block receptors on the detrusor muscle, reducing contractions and making the bladder more stable. They have little effect on cardiac function, but can cause drowsiness and confusion in elderly people; other side effects include dry mouth, constipation and blurred vision.
• Tolterodine has less effect on salivary gland receptors, so dry mouth is less common.
• Imipramine, a tricyclic antidepressant, has anticholinergic and anti-α-adrenoceptor activity; it may be useful in bladder stabilization and nocturia.
• Desmopressin (DDAVP) is an analogue of vasopressin, which reduces the production of urine by up to 50%. Taken intranasally at night it reduces nocturia.

Persistent incontinence

If the incontinence cannot be eliminated, good containment is essential:
• Pads and pants: expensive; problems with delivery of supplies and disposal of soiled pads.
• Intermittent self-catheterization: patient must be motivated.
• Indwelling catheters may seem like an ideal method, but they predispose to chronic urinary infections, get blocked and limit sex life [2].
• Early liaison with local continence adviser and joining self-help groups.

Complications

Complications of recurrent incontinence are associated with a marked reduction in quality of life, and include:
• unpleasant smell and discomfort
• skin irritation and maceration leading to pressure sores
• loss of self-esteem and reluctance to go out, leading to social isolation, loss of fitness, depression and sexual problems—all contribute to a marked decrease in the quality of life
• increased burden on carers (extra washing), making it more difficult for affected people to remain in their own home.

Information for patients

Patients could be referred to the Continence Society [5].

2.4.2 FAECAL INCONTINENCE

• Common with advancing age.
• Very common in the setting of a residential or nursing home [6].
• A frequent reason for institutionalization.

Aetiology

In frail elderly people, common causes include the following:
• Overflow diarrhoea secondary to high constipation
• Sudden severe diarrhoea of any cause in an immobile patient
• Dementia.
  In the general population, common causes include:
• Damage to the anal sphincters during vaginal delivery, especially if the baby was large or forceps were used
• Structural causes, including rectal prolapse and anal fistula
• Damage to the sphincters during anal surgery, e.g. repair of chronic anal fissure, or rarely haemorrhoidectomy
• Neurological causes such as stroke, multiple sclerosis and spinal cord lesions, and loss of sensation secondary to diabetes.

Epidemiology

Faecal incontinence affects:
• 1% of the general population
• 15% of those aged over 85 years living at home
• 10–60% of residents in care homes [7].

Physical signs

Perform a general examination, a rectal examination to assess presence of hard, impacted stool and to assess anal tone, and a neurological assessment if appropriate.

Investigations

Basic blood tests including thyroid function are needed. Specific tests include:
• abdominal film to exclude high constipation
• manometry
• anal endosonography.

Treatment

The following options may be helpful:
• Treat overflow diarrhoea. Explain! If it is the first time the patient or family has encountered this problem, they will be very puzzled by your prescription of laxatives
• Trial of regular toileting

- Behavioural therapy (not evidence based)
- Codeine phosphate or loperamide with bulking agents and regular enemas
- Rarely, there is a case for colostomy in patients with intractable incontinence who want to have more freedom.

Complications

- Social isolation.
- Risk of institutionalization.
- Macerated skin and risk of pressure sores.
- Risk of transmission of intestinal infections, such as *Clostridium difficile* [8].

1 Burgio KL, Mathew KA, Engel BT. Prevalence, incidence and correlates of urinary incontinence in healthy, middle-aged women. *J Urol* 1992; 146: 1255–1259.
2 Saint S, Lipsky BA. Preventing catheter-related bacteriuria. Should we? Can we? How? *Arch Intern Med* 1999; 159: 800–808.
3 Dawson C, Whitfield H. Urinary incontinence and urinary infection. *BMJ* 1996; 312: 961–964.
4 Wise BG, Cardozo LD. Urinary urgency in women. *Br J Hosp Med* 1993; 50: 243–250.
5 Continence Society website: www.vois.org.uk/cf
6 Peet SM, Castleden CM, McGrowther CW. Prevalence of urinary and faecal incontinence in hospitals and residential and nursing homes for older people. *BMJ* 1995; 311: 1063–1064.
7 Royal College of Physicians of London. Incontinence: causes, management and provision of services. *J R Coll Physicians Lond* 1995: 1–5.
8 Wall PG, Ryan MJ. Faecal incontinence in hospitals and residential and nursing homes for elderly people. *BMJ* 1996; 312: 378.
MA Kamm. Fortnightly review: faecal incontinence. *BMJ* 1998; 316: 528–532.

2.5 Hypothermia

Hypothermia occurs, by definition, when the core temperature of the body falls below 35°C.

Aetiology

Except in cases of cold exposure, hypothermia is usually multifactorial with an interaction of ageing changes, disease processes and social factors. Risk factors include:

- old age
- autonomic dysfunction, e.g. diabetes mellitus
- immobility, e.g. cerebrovascular disease (may also affect hypothalamic regulation), Parkinson's disease, rheumatoid arthritis, etc.
- falls
- hypothyroidism (reduced metabolic rate, drowsiness, poor mobility, apathy)
- alcohol
- cognitive impairment (Alzheimer's disease and multi-infarct dementia both cause damage to central thermoregulation and the normal behavioural adjustments to cold are absent)
- drugs that cause vasodilatation, e.g. phenothiazines, calcium antagonists
- poor socioeconomic conditions, e.g. no central heating, and poor clothing and insulation.

Pathophysiology

There is impairment of thermoregulation with ageing. The hypothalamus is thought to act in a similar fashion to a thermostat. In response to cold, the hypothalamus triggers mechanisms of peripheral vasoconstriction, shivering and piloerection via the autonomic nervous system. Changes in the autonomic nervous system with ageing, chiefly a reduction in receptor sensitivity, result in a reduced response to sympathetic and parasympathetic nerve stimulation. The metabolic rate is also reduced in old age which reduces heat generation. These changes reduce the homeostatic response to cold.

Epidemiology

Studies estimate that 10% of people living at home who are aged over 75 years have core body temperatures of <35°C and 1–3% of all patients admitted to hospital in the winter are hypothermic.

Clinical presentation

Patients are often found at home alone on the floor following a fall. Confusion, hallucinations and paranoid features can occur.

Physical signs

Patients are pale and cold to the touch and consciousness is impaired. The core body temperature taken rectally with a low-range thermometer is <35°C (oral readings are inaccurate). There is a bradycardia and hypotension. There may be evidence of pneumonia or pulmonary oedema (caused by cardiac suppression and bradycardia). Muscles are generally rigid and speech may be slurred. There may be signs of a stroke that could have precipitated hypothermia. Also be alert for signs of hypothyroidism, which may be a precipitating cause.

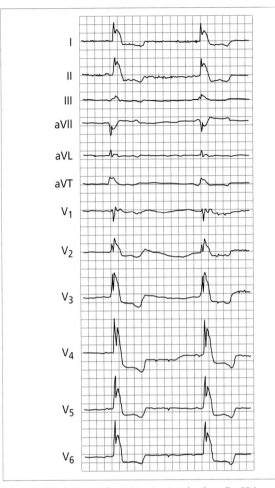

used with caution and a urinary catheter is needed for accurate measurement of urine output. Antibiotics are often needed, because pulmonary infection is common. Underlying disease, e.g. hypothyroidism, should be treated.

Complications

An important complication of hypothermia is pancreatitis: epigastric pain, shock and the consequences of hypocalcaemia.

Prognosis

The mortality rate varies between 30% and 80%.

Prevention

Prevention is better than cure! Campaigns are run to increase public awareness; elderly people are encouraged to have good home heating and insulation, electric blankets and sufficient clothing, and those at risk need regular visits, e.g. to provide hot food.

 Hanania NA, Zimmerman JL. Accidental hypothermia. *Crit Care Clin* 1999; 15: 235–249.
Lloyd EL. Accidental hypothermia. *Resuscitation* 1996; 32: 111–124.

Fig. 14 ECG changes in hypothermia: sinus bradycardia, PR interval 0.2 s. Broad slurred J waves are seen adjacent to the initial QRS deflection in all leads, but most obviously in leads I, II and V2–V6. There is pronounced ST segment depression and T-wave inversion. (This ECG was kindly provided by Dr Derek J Rowlands, Consultant Cardiologist from his text *Understanding the Electrocardiogram:* section 2: morphological abnormalities. Copyright ICI plc 1982.)

Investigations

Baseline investigations should be organized: full blood count, electrolytes, blood glucose, calcium, amylase and thyroid function tests, chest radiograph and ECG. The ECG may show a variety of abnormalities (Fig. 14).

Treatment

The patient should be re-warmed slowly (0.5–1°C per hour) in a warm room and covered with a blanket or 'Bair hugger'—a device through which warm air is blown. Foil blankets are 'out'—they keep the cold in! Rapid re-warming increases mortality as a result of sudden hypotension from vasodilatation and cardiac arrhythmias. Cardiac monitoring is necessary so that arrhythmias (most commonly ventricular tachycardia and ventricular fibrillation when the temperature reaches 31–33°C) can be treated. Intravenous fluids should be

2.6 Drugs in elderly people

General points

Elderly people consume most medications (remember prescribed and OTC drugs). Older people:
• are more sensitive to drugs (often have low weight, reduced renal clearance, decreased hepatic blood flow, etc.)
• are more susceptible to side effects and adverse effects
• have side effects that are more likely to have serious sequelae.
See *Clinical pharmacology*, Section 4.

 Case history example

Nellie Smith doesn't get out much because of her arthritic knees (think vitamin D deficiency and lack of fitness). She is prescribed an NSAID and gets indigestion, but decides this is normal at her age. She has a haematemesis. Blood loss that would be tolerated in a younger person causes collapse because of diminished homeostasis. She fractures her hip (osteoporosis). She lives alone, so she is not found until the next day. She is admitted, but has renal failure (blood loss, unable to get water, poor renal-concentrating ability, the NSAID and her furosemide (frusemide)), and must be 'stabilized' before surgery. Pressure sores worsen, antibiotics are prescribed and she develops *Clostridium difficile* diarrhoea. You can predict the outcome. Was the NSAID indicated initially?

Multiple pathology means multiple therapy and a greater likelihood that a drug will be contraindicated. Older people on several drugs are likely to:
• experience drug interactions (the numbers of drugs and increased sensitivity to each)
• have problems with compliance, especially if confused.

Writing up or reviewing a drug chart

Review your patient's problem list and prioritize the treatable. The patient is usually on many drugs already.

Drug considerations

• Still indicated? (would a non-drug alternative be as effective; has the situation changed, e.g. stop oxybutynin if the patient is incontinent despite it)
• Do likely benefits outweigh risks? (if the patient is only 71 but has dementia, is prone to falls and is admitted with an international normalized ratio (INR) of 7.2, replace warfarin for atrial fibrillation with aspirin)
• 'Nicest' drug for the job? (clarithromycin instead of erythromycin)
• Cheapest? (if there are equivalents, e.g. H_2-receptor blockers)
• Is the drug causing the symptoms? (nausea or confusion as a result of codeine)
• Could a single agent replace two? (ACE inhibitor for hypertension with congestive heart failure)
• Is the formulation/route of administration the best? (syrups and patches may help)
• Timings appropriate? (once or twice daily options aid compliance, especially if drugs are given by visiting carers)
• Aids to administration? (spacer for inhalers, avoid child-proof tops)
• Aids to compliance? (Dosette box)
• Regular or 'as required'? (analgesics for chronic pain are usually best given on a regular basis)
• Does the patient understand the medications and any precautions? (provide written information and record advice given, e.g. for a sore throat on carbimazole, in the notes)
• Should a new drug be started? A drug may be considered for cure or disease modification, symptom control or primary or secondary prevention.

• When prescribing, start low and go slow, but increase the dose until it is in the probable therapeutic range or side effects develop.
• Give a drug for long enough before deciding it is ineffective (e.g. antidepressants).
• If problems arise and a drug is stopped, record this (e.g. ACE inhibitor led to hypotension).
• In prevention, it is particularly important to consider the overall burden of pathology and drugs, but avoid therapeutic nihilism.

Overall picture

• If there are multiple drugs, is everything essential?
• Try to avoid prescribing a drug to treat the side effects of another (e.g. furosemide (frusemide) and fludrocortisone).
• Look for potential interactions.
• If the patient has renal or hepatic failure, don't rely on memory, check every drug against the lists in the BNF (*British National Formulary*). Check if your hospital subscribes to the BNF on-line.
• Use generic names unless bioavailability is crucial or when using a slow-release preparation.
• The patient will change. Always review medication.

Never write up drugs from a GP letter when you are not sure what they are!

British National Formulary. Section on prescribing for the elderly. London: British Medical Association and the Royal Pharmaceutical Society of Great Britain.

2.7 Dementia

Perhaps being old is having lighted rooms inside your head, and people in them, acting. People you know, yet can't quite name.
(Philip Larkin)

Dementia is a syndrome (lots of causes) of acquired (not congenital), chronic (lasts months to years), global (not just memory or just language problems) impairment of higher brain function, in an alert patient (not drowsy), which interferes with the ability to cope with daily living.
It doesn't usually matter if an old person doesn't know 'it's Tuesday', but if she doesn't know 'it's winter' she might freeze. Presentation depends on familiarity and complexity of the environment, as well as on cognition.

Aetiology

The common primary dementias (i.e. the disease mainly affects the brain) in old age are Alzheimer's disease, dementia in Parkinson's disease and Lewy body disease [1,2] (see *Psychiatry*, Section 2.2 and *Neurology*, Section 2.7). The most common secondary dementia is vascular dementia, which includes multiple small infarcts and white matter ischaemia.

DEMENTIA—an acronym for those with poor memories!
*D*rugs and alcohol
*E*yes and ears
*M*etabolic (thyroid)
*E*motional (really, psychiatric problems)
*N*utritional (vitamin B$_{12}$ and other vitamin deficiencies)
*T*rauma and tumours
*I*nfections (syphilis and HIV)
*A*theroma (vascular dementia).

Epidemiology

Dementia is rare below 55 years of age, but the prevalence increases dramatically with age to about 2% in the over-65s and 20% in the over-80s. In elderly people, Alzheimer's disease probably accounts for around two-thirds of cases. Demographic changes are resulting in marked increases in the numbers of the very old and dementia is a major cause of dependency and institutional care. The cost of health and social care for patients with Alzheimer's disease in England [3] has been estimated at over £1 billion (1992–93 prices).

Clinical presentation

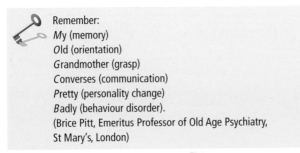 Remember:
*M*y (memory)
*O*ld (orientation)
*G*randmother (grasp)
*C*onverses (communication)
*P*retty (personality change)
*B*adly (behaviour disorder).
(Brice Pitt, Emeritus Professor of Old Age Psychiatry, St Mary's, London)

Postoperative or acute confusion may reflect 'decreased brain reserve' and may predict later dementia. The onset of dementia is usually insidious with gradual changes in memory, thinking processes, language use, personality, behaviour and orientation. Families report that it can be difficult to obtain a diagnosis. If the patient lives alone, there may be no one to give a history and, unless cognition is tested, it is easy to be misled by 'a good social front'. The condition progresses to obvious problems with short-term memory and basic activities of daily living, increasing disorientation and sometimes difficult or distressing behaviour. Eventually, the patient ceases to communicate and becomes totally dependent. Dementia may present acutely, e.g. with the death of the caring spouse.

There is no antemortem diagnostic test for most of the primary dementias, so the likely cause is determined by the clinical features and investigations. Progressive deterioration is common in Alzheimer's disease, whereas step-wise deterioration is characteristic of vascular dementia. Neuropsychiatric phenomena such as delusions and hallu-cinations and extreme sensitivity to major tranquillizers are a feature of Lewy body disease. Parkinsonian features on examination suggest vascular dementia or Lewy body disease. Common conditions such as vascular dementia and Alzheimer's disease may coexist.

Physical signs

A mental state examination is essential (including mood). Record a recognized score, e.g. MMSE (Mini-Mental State Examination). The general state of the patient (signs of neglect) reflects the severity of the management problem. Focus on the neurological and cardiovascular systems, but physical signs may be absent. Other unreported pathology may be found.

Investigations

Investigations typically include blood tests to exclude reversible causes or other major pathology (full blood count, biochemical profile, ESR, thyroid function, vitamin B$_{12}$, folate), chest radiograph, ECG and CT brain scan.

Differential diagnosis

Many old people are slightly forgetful and it can be difficult to distinguish ageing changes from early dementia. The differential diagnosis includes acute confusion (delirium), depression, communication difficulties caused by deafness, poor vision or language deficits, Parkinson's disease, schizophrenia and mania. In an acute confusional state consciousness is impaired. A person can become delirious at any age, but frail older people often become confused when they are ill. The confusion may resolve with the illness or merely improve if there is underlying dementia. Depression may be overlooked or missed in elderly people, may mimic dementia (pseudo-dementia), and may be more common in dementia for pathological and psychological reasons.

Treatment

 Management depends on severity and whether the patient lives alone. It requires a multidisciplinary, multiagency package of care, which is co-ordinated and evolves as the needs of the patient and carer change.

Management options include the following:
- Coping strategies and psychological techniques
- Optimize hearing and vision, and improve general health
- Treat other conditions that may impair cognition (e.g. anaemia, heart failure)
- Education and support for carers (essential—see below)

• Genetic counselling (not indicated for patients or family in dementia in old age)

• Legal advice (e.g. an Enduring Power of Attorney may obviate the need for the Court of Protection at a later date (see Section 2.13, p. 92), advice about driving, advance directives, etc.)

• Therapy assessments (occupational therapy, speech and language therapy—swallowing and communication—and physiotherapy: the aim is usually assessment to plan care and advise carers, rather than treat the patient)

• Assessment by social services (financial entitlements, especially Attendance Allowance, provision of services such as home help and access to 'care management'—the process by which frail old people are assessed for substantial packages of care at home or residential care)

• District nurse/community psychiatric nurse support

• Sitting services (Crossroads), day hospital, respite care

• Proper provision of long-term care

• Drugs may be used:

–for secondary prevention (e.g. aspirin and anti-hypertensives to try to slow progression in vascular dementia)

–to treat specific symptoms and behaviours (major tranquillizers, unfortunately, often the only option)

–to enhance cholinergic transmission in Alzheimer's disease because cholinergic neurons bear the brunt of the damage. Acetylcholinesterase inhibitors (e.g. donepezil and rivastigmine) have some efficacy [4], but there is debate about the extent of clinical benefit.

Complications

Dementia is devastating for the patient and the family. In the late stages the patient is debilitated, doubly incontinent and bed-bound.

Prognosis

In addition to the considerable morbidity, Alzheimer's disease is the fourth leading cause of death in the West. The prognosis depends on the pathology, age and support that the patient receives.

Prevention

Nothing has been proven to prevent Alzheimer's disease. Avoid head injuries and risk factors for vascular disease. Possibilities include keeping the brain active, anti-inflammatory agents, antioxidants and oestrogen (hormone replacement therapy).

Disease associations

Other illnesses may not be reported and the carer may become depressed and neglect his or her physical illnesses.

Important information for patients/carers

Carers need considerable support. The Alzheimer's Disease Society deals with other dementias too and produces excellent literature. The Carers' National Association supports carers in all settings.

1 Small GW, Rabins PV, Barry PP *et al*. Diagnosis and treatment of Alzheimer disease and related disorders. Consensus statement of the American Association for Geriatric Psychiatry, the Alzheimer's Association, and the American Geriatrics Society. *JAMA* 1997; 278: 1363–1371.

2 St George-Hyslop PH. Molecular genetics of Alzheimer's disease. *Biol Psychiatry* 2000; 47: 183–199.

3 Gray A, Fenn P. Alzheimer's disease: the burden of illness in England. *Health Trends* 1993; 25: 331–337.

4 Cummings JL. Cholinesterase inhibitors: a new class of psychotropic compounds. *Am J Psychiatry* 2000; 157: 4–15.

An excellent scientific website is available at
http://www.alzforum.org/members/index
Practical information is available at
http://www.alzheimers.org.uk

2.8 Rehabilitation

Learn to distinguish between impairment, disability and handicap.

Definitions

• Rehabilitation: the process by which an individual attains his or her maximum physical, mental and social capability [1,2].

• Impairment: an objective reduction in physical or mental ability of an individual caused by disease or disorder and which may be temporary or permanent.

• Disability: the effect that the impairment has on daily function.

• Handicap: the disadvantage within society that results from impairment or disability.

• Activities of daily living: ADLs are the functional abilities that a person needs to live independently, e.g. washing, dressing, shopping, cooking, etc.

Case history example

A 76-year-old man has a hemiplegia following a stroke. The grade 3–4 weakness affecting his left side is the impairment. This results in disability, e.g. he is unable to walk independently. The handicap he experiences will depend on his previous lifestyle, but would include not being able to get out to the pub or taking his wife dancing.

Epidemiology

The number of disabled people is increasing as the population is ageing. This reflects the increased prevalence of disabling conditions in old age, e.g. stroke, cardiorespiratory disease, blindness and arthritis. About 4.3 million people aged over 60 years in Britain are disabled and 90% live in their own homes.

Rehabilitation

The team

Rehabilitation is an active and energetic process and involves a team, the patient being a member of the team and at its centre. The other members of the multidisciplinary team are: the doctor (usually a geriatrician), nurses, physiotherapists, occupational therapists, speech and language therapists, and a medical social worker. Other members who may be approached as appropriate include a podiatrist (chiropodist), psychologist, continence adviser and dietitian.

The setting

Rehabilitation can be performed anywhere, but it is usual to have a dedicated unit or ward where staff with appropriate skills are concentrated. Purpose-built units have adequate space around beds and in bathrooms to encourage independence. Patients need space to store their belongings because they will usually be up and dressed in their own clothes. There are usually large day room and dining areas for social activities. The physiotherapy gym and occupational therapy department (with bedroom and kitchen) are part of the unit. The doctor's role is to determine pathology and impairments, i.e. diagnosis, and often to co-ordinate the team.

The process

The process of rehabilitation is usually focused on setting appropriate short- and longer-term goals. The goals must be realistic, so it is essential to know what the patient could do before the current episode and what the patient wants.

Case conferences are usually held weekly to monitor each patient's progress.

Discharge planning

Various ADL scales are used to monitor the patient's progress, e.g. the Barthel Index (see Section 3.2, p. 95). Discharge planning begins at the time of admission. The process is fine-tuned as the patient progresses. An independent flatlet within the unit may be used to monitor a patient's capabilities as the time for discharge approaches. If functional impairment remains, which is often the case, the patient has a 'needs assessment' before discharge. If it is thought that he or she can live in the community, a home visit is carried out by the occupational therapist with his or her spouse/relatives present. This helps determine whether aids and appliances at home would be needed to lessen disability and whether the living environment needs alteration, e.g. widening of doorways for wheelchair access, or the removal of obstacles, such as worn carpets. A social worker is involved in the process to assess need for social care, e.g. home helps for shopping, meals-on-wheels service. The social worker will also assess whether the patient is eligible for benefits, e.g. Attendance Allowance (see Section 2.12, p. 92).

Specialist units

There are also specialized rehabilitation units, e.g. stroke units and orthogeriatric units, which usually have specific protocols for admission. Stroke units have been shown to result in a better outcome for stroke patients in terms of their mortality and functional recovery (see Section 1.4, p. 59). Orthogeriatric units, in which elderly patients with a fractured neck of the femur are under the joint care of an orthopaedic surgeon and geriatrician, enable better provision of perioperative care. There is also early rehabilitation assessment and, if necessary, transfer to the general rehabilitation unit.

Day rehabilitation

Geriatric day hospitals are day rehabilitation units which are within the hospital and run by geriatricians. Patients usually attend 1 or 2 days a week on an outpatient basis. They attend for rehabilitation, maintenance treatment or medical and nursing investigations. In some areas of the country, the day hospital has been replaced by 'outreach rehabilitation teams', where rehabilitation is provided in the patient's own home but is co-ordinated in the hospital by a geriatrician.

If, after the process of rehabilitation, it is apparent that the patient cannot continue to live in his or her own home, residential or nursing home accommodation has to be considered (see Section 1.4, p. 61).

1 Henschke P, Finucane PM. Rehabilitation. In: Pathy MSJ, ed. *Principles and Practice of Geriatric Medicine*, 3rd edn. Chichester: Wiley, 1998: 1403–1416.
2 Young J. Rehabilitation and older people. *BMJ* 1996; 313: 677–681.

2.9 Aids and appliances

Aids and appliances can reduce disability, increase independence and may lessen handicap.

Case history example

Following his rehabilitation programme, a patient has permanent neurological impairment (see Section 2.8, p. 85), but with a tripod and foot splint can walk well enough to get out to his son's car and down to the pub.

A huge range of aids and appliances is available, ranging in price from pence (rubber non-slip mats for plates) to thousands of pounds (stair lifts). Many families buy aids privately and if they are costly should always be encouraged to obtain professional advice before parting with their cash! Occupational therapists assess patients for most of these, with the exception of walking aids for which patients are assessed by a physiotherapist.

A brief summary of some of the most common aids is given below.

Kitchen aids

- Tap turner (Fig. 15): easier to turn taps for those with limb weakness or arthritis.
- Kettle tipper (Fig. 16): useful for tremor, weakness and poor vision.
- Cutlery (Fig. 17): antispill device for the plate for those who have use of one hand, and easy to hold cutlery for weak or arthritic hands.
- Potato peeler (Fig. 18): for a hemiplegic patient.

Dressing aids

- Long-handled shoehorn.
- Much can be achieved by altering the style of dress, e.g. opt for V-necked sweater rather than a cardigan or slip-on shoes rather than lace-ups, or replace fastenings with Velcro.

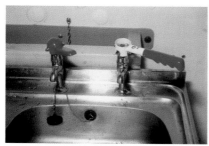

Fig. 15 Tap turner.

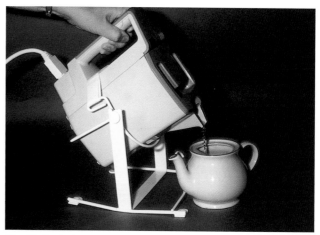

Fig. 16 Kettle tipper.

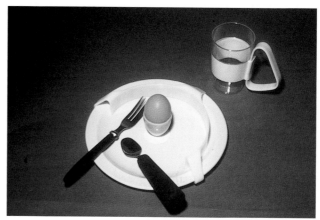

Fig. 17 Cutlery.

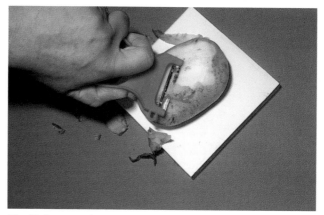

Fig. 18 Potato peeler.

Mobility aids

- Walking sticks: they relieve pain by giving support and aid locomotion. One or two sticks may be required. Many types exist, e.g. single rod, tripods and tetrapods (useful as they remain 'standing' if put down temporarily). Assessment and accurate length measurement are essential.
- Zimmer frames/Rollators: consider the home as well as the person. May need a frame both upstairs and downstairs.

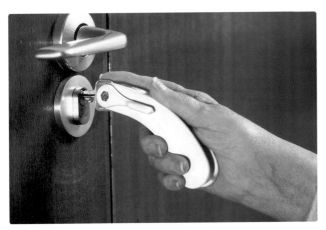

Fig. 19 Key holder.

• Wheelchairs: these are expensive. Correct size, wheel style (push or self-propel) and padding are essential.

Others

• Helping hand.
• Key holder (Fig. 19).
• Pendant alarm: to call for help by pressing pendant, which alerts family/neighbours by remote control.
• High seat chairs.
• Extra stair rails (both sides of a steep flight, adjacent to steps between rooms).
• Raised toilet seat.

Disabled Living Centres are in the phone book.
Information and catalogues for aids for specific conditions are usually most helpful from specialist societies, e.g. RNIB, Stroke Association, Parkinson's Disease Society.
Mulley G, Penn N, Burns E. *Older People at Home: Practical Issues.* London: BMJ Publishing Group, 1998.

2.10 Hearing impairment

• Deafness is very common in elderly people.
• Presbyacusis is the most common cause in the over-70s.
• Always examine the eardrum in any patient with deafness.
• Use a communicator.
• Beware unilateral deafness; think of acoustic neuroma and cholesteatoma.

Aetiology

Conductive deafness may be caused by the following:
• Wax
• A foreign body
• Postinfective mastoiditis

• Chronic suppurative otitis media
• Paget's disease of the skull
• Tumours: glomus tumour, cholesteatoma
• Otosclerosis: a congenital disease, caused by (usually) bilateral replacement of the stapes with spongy non-conducting bone; twice as common in women and 50% have a family history. Management involves stapedectomy with an artificial implant.

Sensorineural deafness is caused by the following:
• Presbyacusis
• Noise-induced damage
• Neurological conditions: acoustic neuroma, Menière's disease (usually middle-aged, not elderly, people), meningioma, multiple sclerosis, stroke
• Ototoxic drugs: aminoglycosides especially gentamicin, loop diuretics, cisplatin, aspirin
• Infections: measles, mumps, meningitis, influenza, herpes, syphilis
• Congenital sensorineural deafness, which may be isolated or part of a syndrome, e.g.:
  –Alport's syndrome—sensorineural deafness and glomerulonephritis
  –Apert's syndrome—sensorineural deafness and acrocephalosyndactyly
  –Usher's syndrome—sensorineural deafness and retinitis pigmentosa.

Epidemiology

• In 60% of those aged over 70 years.
• Of this age group, 25% would benefit from a hearing aid.

Clinical presentation

Usually this is obvious, but deafness may be overlooked as a contributory factor in depression, paranoia, acute confusion and dementia. Coexisting tinnitus may be troublesome.

Physical signs

Always look in the ear canal, mainly for wax but also for cholesteatoma. Tuning fork tests will discriminate between conductive and sensory deafness.
• Rinne's test: normally, air conduction is better than bone conduction so that a positive (normal) Rinne's test is when sound is heard better with the prongs of the tuning fork held near the ear than when the base is placed on the mastoid process.
• Weber's test: the tuning fork is placed on the top of the head, and the test is normal when the sound is detected equally well in both ears.

In unilateral deafness look for signs of a cerebellopontine angle lesion.

Investigations

Refer to the audiology service where a pure-tone audiogram and speech audiogram will be performed. In presbyacusis, the pure-tone audiogram shows that high frequencies are particularly impaired. To record a speech audiogram, a list of sentences is presented under controlled conditions; this gives the best indication of whether a hearing aid will be helpful.

Treatment

General measures

- When talking with people with hearing impairment, make sure that they can see your face and try to reduce background noise or use a communication device.
- To remove wax, first prescribe ear drops to soften it, sodium bicarbonate or olive oil, then refer for syringing.
- Refer to audiology for an assessment for a hearing aid or masker for tinnitus.
- Educate about environmental aids: warning light on telephones, door bells and smoke alarms, vibrating pillows as alarm clocks, subtitles on television and the 'closed caption' system on videos.
- Hospitals flag patients' notes so that clinic staff are aware of hearing impairment.
- An older person may be greatly helped by a hearing dog (see below).

Hearing aids

Many elderly people do not wear their hearing aids. This may be because the aids do not restore normal hearing, because all noises are amplified so that speech especially is difficult to hear, and because of feedback problems (the loud whistling associated with hearing aids) and the attached stigma.

To get the best from a hearing aid:
- encourage the new wearer to use it regularly early on to get used to it
- ensure that the ear mould fits well and is comfortable
- make sure that the patient is able to fit it him- or herself
- the batteries should be live and it should be switched on!
- wax should not be allowed to build up in the ear canals
- arrange regular follow-up and support
- explain use of the 'T' position (an induction loop) with adapted telephones, ticket offices, theatres, etc.

For the future

Digital hearing aids will be used more widely because they can amplify speech frequency and reduce background noise and there is less feedback. Implantable hearing aids also reduce feedback and improve speech clarity. Centres in the USA are offering cochlear implants to elderly people and have excellent outcomes.

Complications

Deafness is more disabling than it appears.
- Social isolation because of reduced ability to communicate.
- Impaired sense of balance and increased falls.
- Increased risk of accidents because of lack of audible cues (car horns, warning shouts).
- Potential for confusion (and paranoia) when admitted to hospital. Try the hints above.

Patient information

Make the patient aware of:
- Hearing Concern [1]
- Royal National Institute for Deaf People (RNID) website [2]
- Hearing dogs [3].

Mills R. The auditory system. In: Pathy MSJ, ed. *Principles and Practice of Geriatric Medicine*, 3rd edn. Chichester: Wiley, 1998: 1093–1104.
1 Hearing Concern website: http://www.hearingconcern.com
2 Royal National Institute for Deaf People website: http://www.ucl.ac.uk/Library/RNID/rnid.htm
3 Hearing dogs website: http://www.hearing-dogs.co.uk

2.11 Nutrition

Thousands are annually starved in the midst of plenty for want alone of the means to take food. (Florence Nightingale)
Although Florence Nightingale's patients were considerably younger, many older people today are poorly nourished both at home and (particularly) in institutions.

Aetiology

Malnutrition is usually multifactorial with contributions from the consequences of ageing, social factors and pathology [1]. Key factors include:
- socioeconomic deprivation (social isolation and/or poverty)
- poor oral hygiene/dentition
- mental illness
- physical illness
- iatrogenic.

Mental illness

Depression causes anorexia and apathy and, in severe cases, food refusal. Bereavement may remove the social aspects of eating. Undernutrition in Alzheimer's disease is not fully understood, but decreased food intake and increased energy expenditure as a result of agitation contribute.

Physical illness

A number of conditions make food preparation difficult. Illness may cause anorexia and nausea, resulting in a reduced energy intake. There may be swallowing problems, e.g. stroke, or malabsorption, for which there are many causes, e.g. inflammatory bowel disease, coeliac disease and small bowel bacterial overgrowth, all of which are not uncommon in elderly people. Protein may be lost via the kidney, gut or skin, and energy expenditure may be increased, e.g. in infection.

Iatrogenic

• Drugs causing: anorexia, e.g. digoxin; altered taste, e.g. ACE inhibitors; dry mouth and nausea, e.g. specific SSRIs; and constipation, e.g. opiates.
• Special diets or food textures, e.g. low-salt diets or thickened foods are often unpalatable.

Causes are often multiple. Cardiac cachexia (Fig. 20), for example, is defined as undernutrition occurring as a consequence of congestive heart failure. Its aetiology is multifactorial and includes: decreased intake as a result of anorexia caused by breathlessness, drugs, gastric and liver congestion, an increased metabolic rate and malabsorption. A similar situation occurs in many cancers.

Epidemiology

Undernutrition is common in elderly people and causes substantial morbidity and mortality. Large community nutritional surveys have been completed since the 1960s. The National Diet and Nutrition Survey, commissioned by the Ministry of Agriculture, Fisheries and Food and the Department of Health in 1995, assessed people aged over 65 years—1275 living at home and 412 in institutions [2]. Some of its conclusions are as follows:
• There is a strong correlation between diet, nutritional status and oral health
• Energy intakes for those living at home were lower than estimated average requirements
• Average fibre intake was below the average recommended levels in both groups
• Average intakes of vitamins A, B_6, D and folate were below the recommended level
• Those of low socioeconomic status had lower intakes of energy, protein, carbohydrate, fibre and vitamins (especially vitamin C)
• Low body weight, defined as a body mass index of 20 kg/m^2 or less, was particularly common in those in institutions (3% men and 6% women at home; 16% men and 15% women in institutions).

Physical signs

Clinical features vary but may include the following:
• Signs of protein undernutrition: muscle wasting, peripheral oedema and leuconychia are signs of hypoalbuminaemia
• Signs of anaemia (pallor, angular stomatitis, glossitis, brittle nails)
• Vitamin K deficiency—superficial bruises, oral haemorrhages
• Vitamin D deficiency—osteomalacia may present with proximal myopathy, bone pain, pathological fracture and tetany
• Vitamin C deficiency—petechial and perifollicular haemorrhages, corkscrew hairs, mucosal haemorrhages (bleeding gums), gum hypertrophy and haemarthroses
• Vitamin B_{12} deficiency—peripheral neuropathy, subacute combined degeneration of the cord, dementia and optic atrophy.

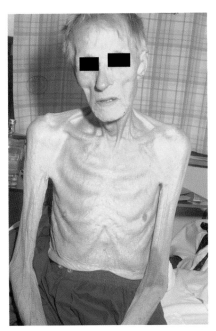

Fig. 20 Severe cachexia with loss of body fat and lean body mass in a patient with cardiac cachexia resulting from mitral valve disease.

 Remember, the obese woman who lives on tea and toast or even sweet sherry may have severe protein and vitamin deficiencies!

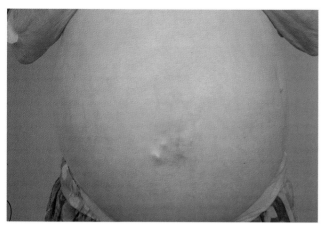

Fig. 21 Gross abdominal distension caused by ascites. There is also caput medusae and the patient has had the umbilicus removed after surgery for an umbilical hernia. The cause is portal hypertension resulting from hepatic cirrhosis.

Signs of underlying cause

These are abdominal distension resulting from ascites caused by hepatic cirrhosis (Fig. 21) and hepatomegaly resulting from malignancy. There may be other signs of chronic liver disease, e.g. finger clubbing, palmar erythema, spider naevi, Dupuytren's contracture, etc. Abdominal distension may be the result of malabsorption, e.g. coeliac disease, inflam-matory bowel disease and small bowel bacterial overgrowth.

Investigations

Document the weight (surprisingly difficult in hospital), noting whether this is distorted by oedema. Refer to the dietitian who will calculate the body mass index (BMI: weight [kg] divided by height [m] squared or calculated from the demi-span if the patient cannot stand), assess previous diet and recommend treatment. Refer for speech and language therapy if dysphagia is a problem. Other investigations depend on the clinical picture.

 Check for hypercalcaemia in nauseated patients with cancer.

Treatment

A multidisciplinary multifaceted approach is most likely to be successful:
• Work with nursing staff, relatives, hospital catering and dietetics to try to provide nutritious, appetizing food and make sure that it is served in a way that ensures that patients eat as much as they are able; snacks should be available
• Ensure that the patient has comfortable dentures

• Treat the underlying causes of poor nutrition
• Review the drug chart
• Improve symptom control, especially a sore mouth, nausea, reflux, pain control, constipation or diarrhoea
• Consider a little alcohol; low-dose steroids may help in some cancers
• Dietary supplements, e.g. Fortisips, Ensure or specific vitamins
• Consider non-oral feeding if indicated, e.g. nasogastric or percutaneous endoscopic gastrostomy feeding or parenteral nutrition, if the gut is not functioning but is expected to recover
• At home, liaise with social services to arrange a luncheon club, provision of meals on wheels or frozen meals, etc.

Complications

Malnutrition is associated with considerable morbidity and has been estimated to cost the health service millions of pounds. Consequences include the following:
• Falls and their sequelae, e.g. fractured neck of femur
• Reduced immunity [3] resulting in recurrent infections, e.g. oral candidiasis (Fig. 22)
• Pressure sores and slow wound healing
• Loss of independence
• Depression and a vicious circle of anorexia and poor nutrition.

Prognosis

In old age, a low BMI is associated with a poor prognosis. Obesity may increase morbidity, e.g. from angina or osteo-arthritic knees, but is not associated with increased mortality in population studies.

Prevention

Identify at-risk patients on the post-take round and take immediate action.

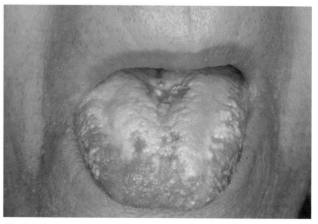

Fig. 22 Oral candidiasis.

1 Vetta F, Ronzoni S, Taglieri G, Bollea MR. The impact of malnutrition on the quality of life in the elderly. *Clin Nutr* 1999; 18: 259–267.

2 Bates CJ, Prentice A, Cole TJ *et al*. Micronutrients: highlights and research challenges from the 1994–5 National Diet and Nutrition Survey of people aged 65 years and over. *Br J Nutr* 1999; 82: 7–15. (References other papers from this survey.)

3 Lesourd B, Mazari L. Nutrition and immunity in the elderly. *Proc Nutr Soc* 1999; 58: 685–695.

Remember people die from severe cardiac failure and lung disease, as well as from cancer.

2.12 Benefits

In general, elderly people have low incomes and being poor correlates strongly with ill health. You are not expected to know all the benefits available, but it is your responsibility to inform patients that there is help available and to direct them to sources of information such as the Citizens Advice Bureau or Age Concern. However, your patients (and possibly even your family) will benefit if you know about the key benefits listed here.

Attendance Allowance (including that for terminal care) is not means tested and is not taxable, so older people are more easily persuaded to apply for it.

Attendance Allowance

This is the equivalent of Disability Living Allowance for those aged under 65 years who need help with mobility and personal hygiene.

• This is money available to a person who:
  –is aged 65 years and over;
  –is physically or mentally ill or disabled; and
  –who needs help with activities of daily living, especially washing, dressing and personal care.

• It is available whether or not he or she lives alone.

• It is paid at two rates, depending on whether the person needs help just in the day or also at night.

Attendance Allowance under the Special Rules

• This is money set aside for people who have a terminal illness with an estimated prognosis of 6 months or less, even if they are completely independent.

• It can be applied for on the patient's behalf on a very simple form without telling the patient the prognosis.

• The money does not have to be used to pay for care, but to improve the quality of life for the last few months, e.g. to pay for heating, microwave food or taxis to hospital.

Invalid Care Allowance

The Invalid Care Allowance is paid to the carer who looks after someone (who is usually already claiming for Attendance Allowance) for at least 35 hours a week. It should be applied for before the carer reaches 65 years of age. It is not income related, but is not paid if the carer is earning more than £50 a week from employment after allowable expenses, and may affect other benefits. The sum is not large, but the carer will usually be credited with National Insurance contributions, which protect the basic retirement pension.

Age Concern Factsheet 34: Attendance Allowance and Disability Living Allowance. Age Concern, 1999. Benefits Agency website: www.dss.gov.uk/ba

2.13 Legal aspects of elderly care

Mental capacity

A lack of mental capacity may arise because someone is unable to make a decision because of his or her mental state, because he or she cannot communicate that decision, or a combination of the two [1].

A person's capacity may vary depending on the nature of the decision, and fluctuate from day to day. If a person has communication problems, an attempt must be made to overcome the difficulties before concluding that the person does not have the capacity.

The question is 'does the person understand the nature and likely consequence of the decision that needs to be made, and can they communicate this'?

Testamentary capacity

People who are confused or have mental health problems may still have testamentary capacity (be able to make a valid will). They must be aware that a will is being made, have a reasonable grasp of the nature and extent of their assets and the relationship of the possible beneficiaries, and be able to communicate their wishes. Assessment of testamentary capacity should include standard tests of cognitive function, e.g. Mini-Mental State Examination, but it is often more helpful to ask directly about the family members and whether the patient owns his or her house, where it is, etc.

Power of Attorney

This is a legal document where a person (the donor) enables another (known as the attorney, but usually a family member, not a solicitor) to act on his or her behalf. It is restricted to financial matters [2]. The donor must have capacity (as described above) to make it valid. The donor directs the attorney. However, if the donor becomes mentally incompetent, the Power of Attorney ceases and the Court of Protection has to be contacted to take over the donor's financial affairs.

Enduring Power of Attorney

This is a Power of Attorney that endures, i.e. is still legally effective even if the donor becomes mentally incompetent. It was introduced in England and Wales in 1985. Scottish law is different—a Power of Attorney made after 1 January 1991 is still lawful, even if the donor becomes mentally incompetent, providing the donor has not stated otherwise.

 If you suspect that a patient has a dementing illness, do raise the subject of an Enduring Power of Attorney at an early stage with the spouse or children. It is a simple, cheap procedure. If it is not applied for, once the patient loses capacity, there is no alternative but direct application to the Court of Protection which is expensive and cumbersome.

When an attorney believes that the donor has become mentally incompetent, the Enduring Power of Attorney has to be registered with the Court of Protection for which there is a fee. The Court of Protection can terminate an Enduring Power of Attorney if the attorney becomes mentally incapable or is found to be dishonest.

The Court of Protection

This exists to supervise the management of the financial affairs of those who are mentally incapable. It can write or change a will as appropriate for a patient. Referral to the Court of Protection can be made by a relative, friend or doctor, etc. when an Enduring Power of Attorney does not exist. A doctor (the patient's GP or consultant) is asked to complete a medical certificate stating that the patient is incapable of managing his or her affairs as a result of mental disorder. The Court charges a commencement fee, then an annual fee and a fee for any transaction that the Court authorizes, e.g. for sale of a house.

Living Wills or Advance Directives

A person of sound mind can state that, if certain circumstances arise in the future and he or she becomes mentally and/or physically incapacitated from a serious illness, certain treatment should or should not occur. Advance directives have force in common law. There must be evidence that they were completed and witnessed when the subject was in sound mind and not depressed and he or she fully understood the nature of the directions.

Elder abuse

Elder abuse was first described in Britain in 1975. In the USA there is a legal requirement to notify the authorities of suspected cases, but this is not so at present in Britain. However, hospitals now have elder abuse policies and police stations have officers with special responsibility for elder abuse. Studies show that 5% of elderly people experience abuse from carers [3].

 There are several forms of elder abuse:
- physical (hitting, restraining)
- psychological
- verbal
- general neglect (deprivation of food, clothing, warmth, etc.)
- financial
- sexual
- misuse of medication, e.g. withholding antianginal drugs, oversedation.

The abuser is often the immediate carer. Abuse is more likely if the patient is immobile, incontinent or mentally impaired, or there were poor family relationships before the caring became necessary. Awareness of elder abuse is the first step to management. Suspicions should be aroused if there are unexplained bruises or falls, or if there is excessive alcohol consumption by the carer. The patient often appears frightened and the carer may exhibit anger or despair. If suspected, the patient and carer must be interviewed alone. The carer must be told of concerns and the case referred to a social worker for continued monitoring. If abuse is in a residential or nursing home, the relevant inspection body has to be informed immediately. If there is fraud or identifiable injury, the police should be informed with the agreement of the patient if he or she is mentally competent.

1 Miller SS, Marin DB. Assessing capacity. *Emerg Med Clin North Am* 2000; 18: 233–242.
2 Letts P. *Managing Other People's Money*. London: Age Concern, 1990.
3 Bennet G, Kingston P. *Elder Abuse: Concepts, Theories and Intervention*. London: Chapman & Hall, 1993.
4 *Age Concern Factsheet 22*: Legal arrangements for managing financial affairs. Age Concern, January 2000.

3 Investigations and practical procedures

3.1 Diagnosis vs common sense

Will it be helpful to investigate the problem?

Not all symptoms, abnormal physical findings or results should be investigated. The overall likelihood of doing some good must be considered. However, the decision NOT to investigate should be active, not oversight, and be recorded (e.g. ESR 85 mm/h, myeloma screen negative, decision not to investigate further).

Which investigation?

If investigation is appropriate, which investigation should be chosen? For example, a barium swallow and oesophago-gastroduodenoscopy can both be used to investigate dysphagia but have different risks and advantages. Balance diagnostic yield with acceptability to the patient, risk of the procedure and availability in your hospital. Be aware of costs, but most costs are insignificant compared with delays in discharge.

Is investigation justified?

A diagnostic test may be justified if it helps social management, even if immediate medical management will not change, e.g. an elderly man with confusion, iron deficiency and change in bowel habit is a poor candidate for surgery, so why pursue a diagnosis? An abdominal CT scan is usually well tolerated (unlike a barium enema). A scan highly suggestive of cancer may enable the family to struggle on for another few months without seeking institutional care, knowing that the end is in sight. Support can be arranged from palliative care services and, if a chest infection or acute obstruction supervenes, the GP can arrange terminal care, not urgent admission. Conversely, investigation of risk factors when treatment would not be appropriate is unhelpful and may increase anxiety. In a 91-year-old person who has recovered well from a stroke, carotid endarterectomy would not be carried out, so do not arrange Doppler carotid studies. Patients' views about how far they wish to be investigated must be respected.

3.2 Assessment of cognition, mood and function

Management of an older patient requires more than a medical diagnosis; a holistic approach, which includes evaluation of the person's cognition, mood and functional ability, is essential.

Aspects of mental state and function are best recorded using standardized instruments that have been shown to be valid and repeatable. Without such scores, dementia and depression are often overlooked and typical medical notes give little idea of what the patient can actually do.

Abbreviated Mental Test score

The AMT is the most common quick ward test to identify patients who may have cognitive problems [1].

The Abbreviated Mental Test score

Each question scores one mark and the test is marked out of 10. No half marks are allowed. A score of 6 or below is likely to indicate impaired cognition.

1. Age.
2. Time (to nearest hour).
3. Address for recall at end (e.g. 42 West Street).
4. What year is it?
5. Name of institution.
6. Recognition of two persons (can the patient identify your job and that of a nurse?).
7. Date of birth (day and month).
8. Year of First World War.
9. Name of present monarch.
10. Count backwards from 20 to 1.

A low score on a cognitive test indicates that further assessment is needed. It is often the result of acute or chronic confusion (delirium or dementia), but patients also get a low score if they are deaf, dysphasic, depressed, do not speak English or refuse to answer!

Mini-Mental State Examination

If more time is available, the MMSE, devised by Folstein, is more comprehensive [2]. Cognitive domains tested include orientation, registration of information, attention and calculation, recall, language (naming and repeating), reading, writing, the ability to follow a three-stage command and construction (copying two overlapping pentagons). The MMSE is widely used as a screening tool in population studies and may be used to monitor change and the response to treatment in Alzheimer's disease. Education does affect the score. The maximum is 30 but a score of 30 (or 10 on the AMT) does not rule out dementia (e.g. a barrister may score 30 but have problems at work). A score of 28–30 does not support the diagnosis of dementia, 25–27 is borderline and <25 suggests confusion. Of over-75s in the general population, 13% have scores <25.

Geriatric Depression Score

Depression is common in elderly people. The 15-point GDS [3] is a useful screening tool.

The Geriatric Depression Score

A score indicating depression includes positive and negative answers but, unless you are very stressed, you will be able to work this out! A patient scoring 0–4 is not depressed; a patient scoring 5–15 requires further assessment.
Score 1 point: No to 1, 5, 7, 11, 13; Yes to 2, 3, 4, 6, 8, 9, 10, 12, 14, 15.

1	Are you basically satisfied with your life?	No/Yes
2	Have you dropped many of your activities and interests?	Yes/No
3	Do you feel that your life is empty?	Yes/No
4	Do you often get bored?	Yes/No
5	Are you in good spirits most of the time?	No/Yes
6	Are you afraid that something bad is going to happen to you?	Yes/No
7	Do you feel happy most of the time?	No/Yes
8	Do you often feel helpless?	Yes/No
9	Do you prefer to stay at home, rather than going out and doing new things?	Yes/No
10	Do you feel that you have more problems with memory than most?	Yes/No
11	Do you think it is wonderful to be alive?	No/Yes
12	Do you feel pretty worthless the way you are now?	Yes/No
13	Do you feel full of energy?	No/Yes
14	Do you feel that your situation is hopeless?	Yes/No
15	Do you think that most people are better off than you are?	Yes/No

Barthel Activities of Daily Living Index

This score, devised by a physiotherapist, Barthel, is the most common basic activities of daily living scale [4]. It has limitations—there is a marked ceiling effect (a person could score 20 despite considerable handicap), but it can be scored by a nurse, the score correlates with discharge destination and it is widely used in elderly people.

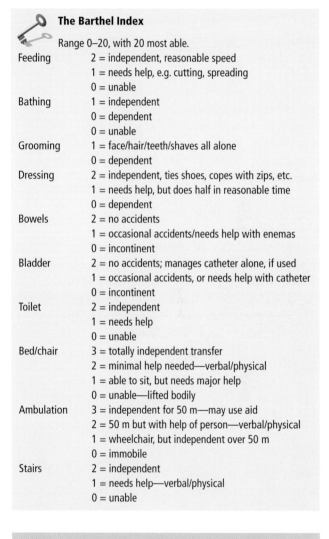

The Barthel Index

Range 0–20, with 20 most able.

Feeding	2 = independent, reasonable speed
	1 = needs help, e.g. cutting, spreading
	0 = unable
Bathing	1 = independent
	0 = dependent
	0 = unable
Grooming	1 = face/hair/teeth/shaves all alone
	0 = dependent
Dressing	2 = independent, ties shoes, copes with zips, etc.
	1 = needs help, but does half in reasonable time
	0 = dependent
Bowels	2 = no accidents
	1 = occasional accidents/needs help with enemas
	0 = incontinent
Bladder	2 = no accidents; manages catheter alone, if used
	1 = occasional accidents, or needs help with catheter
	0 = incontinent
Toilet	2 = independent
	1 = needs help
	0 = unable
Bed/chair	3 = totally independent transfer
	2 = minimal help needed—verbal/physical
	1 = able to sit, but needs major help
	0 = unable—lifted bodily
Ambulation	3 = independent for 50 m—may use aid
	2 = 50 m but with help of person—verbal/physical
	1 = wheelchair, but independent over 50 m
	0 = immobile
Stairs	2 = independent
	1 = needs help—verbal/physical
	0 = unable

1 Hodkinson HM. Evaluation of a mental test score for assessment of mental impairment in the elderly. *Age Ageing* 1972; 1: 233–238.
2 Hope RA, Longmore JM, McManus SK, Wood-Allum CA. *Oxford Handbook of Clinical Medicine*, 4th edn. Oxford: Oxford University Press, 1998: 77.
3 Sheikh JI, Yesavage JA, Brooks JO *et al*. Proposed factor structure of the Geriatric Depression Scale. *Int Psychogeriatr* 1991; 3: 23–28.
4 Coni N, Webster S. *Lecture Notes on Geriatrics*, 5th edn. Oxford: Blackwell Science, 1998: 184.

Answers on pp. 102–104.

Question 1

See Fig. 23. A 75-year-old woman with a history of long-standing rheumatoid arthritis presents with a 2 month history of malaise, during which time she has lost 6 kg of weight. For the last few months her bowels have become a bit erratic, with occasional constipation for which she has had to take a laxative. Her liver is enlarged about 3 finger breadths below the costal margin and feels firm. Examination is otherwise unremarkable. A CT scan of her abdomen is shown (see Fig. 23). The most likely diagnosis is:

A cirrhosis of the liver with ascites
B cirrhosis of the liver
C liver metastases
D liver metastases with ascites
E hepatic amyloidosis

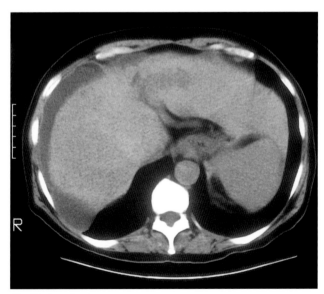

Fig. 23 Question 1.

Question 2

See Fig. 24. A 78-year-old woman is referred with complaints of tiredness, decreasing exercise capacity because of breathlessness, and palpitations. A year ago she had a right-sided stroke, from which she made a reasonable recovery such that she was able to return to her home. She lives alone, is socially isolated and has refused offers of support from social services. A picture of her mouth is shown (see Fig. 24). The most likely diagnosis is:

A scleroderma

B vitamin B12 deficiency
C hereditary haemorrhagic telangiectasia
D coeliac disease
E iron and folate deficiency

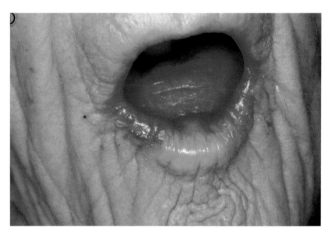

Fig. 24 Question 2.

Question 3

A 74-year-old man has been diagnosed as having idiopathic Parkinson's disease. He is seen in the outpatient clinic and wants to discuss drug treatments available. Which two of the following statements are correct?

A benzhexol has no significant anticholinergic side effects
B benzhexol taken for some time can be stopped abruptly
C benzhexol is especially effective in reducing akinesia
D benzhexol can be safely used in patients with Alzheimer's disease
E amantadine never causes confusion
F levodopa combined with decarboxylase inhibitor crosses the blood/brain barrier
G long term, levodopa may cause dyskinesia and motor fluctuations
H levodopa does not discolour the urine
I apomorphine is a D1 and D2 receptor agonist
J selegiline is a selective inhibitor of monoamine oxidase type A

Question 4

A 74-year-old man is admitted with a history of increasingly poor mobility. Prior to admission he had not been able to get up from his chair. Examination showed bradykinesia, poverty of movement, difficulty in initiating movement and progressive fatiguing and diminishing amplitude of alternating movements. There was no rigidity or tremor, but tone was increased. Which two of the following statements are correct?

A absence of rigidity makes a diagnosis of Parkinson's disease unlikely

B absence of tremor makes a diagnosis of Parkinson's disease unlikely

C the most likely diagnosis is Parkinson's disease

D the cumulative lifetime risk of developing Parkinsonism is 1 in 100

E diagnosis of Parkinson's disease requires extensive laboratory investigation

F diagnosis of Parkinson's disease requires upper body akinesia to be present

G the most likely diagnosis is arteriosclerotic pseudoparkinsonism

H misdiagnosis of Parkinson's disease is uncommon

I cogwheel rigidity does not occur in essential tremor

J rapid progression supports a diagnosis of idiopathic Parkinson's disease

Question 5

A frail 83-year-old man who lives in a nursing home and has type 2 diabetes mellitus is admitted with a chest infection. On general examination you notice that the skin on both heels is pink and boggy. Which statement is true of this situation?

A he is likely to have bilateral deep vein thrombosis

B a minimum 4-hour repositioning schedule should be adopted

C a high carbohydrate diet should be encouraged

D a pressure-relieving support surface should be considered

E there are no validated tools to assess patients at risk of these complications

Question 6

An 87-year-old woman is admitted after being found wandering in her nightie. She says she is looking for her cat. On examination, she smells strongly of alcohol, but is otherwise well. Her medications include paroxetine for depression, lorazepam for anxiety (she is not sure how many she is taking), cimetidine for longstanding peptic ulcer disease and thyroxine 50 mcg daily. Which medication/substance can be stopped immediately without problems?

A paroxetine

B lorazepam

C alcohol

D cimetidine

E thyroxine

Question 7

An 87-year-old woman is admitted to hospital after a fall. She has had four falls over the last 6 weeks. Her medications on admission include amitriptyline 75 mg od, temazepam 20 mg nocte, diazepam 2 mg tds, bendro-fluazide 2.5 mg od, captopril 25 mg tds, ranitidine 150 mg od and amlodipine 10 mg od. Which one of the following statements is correct?

A tapering and discontinuation of benzodiazepines has not been shown to reduce falls

B tapering and discontinuation of tricyclic antidepressants has not been shown to reduce falls

C reducing the total number of medications to 4 or less reduces the risk of falling

D all older patients with postural hypotension are symptomatic

E falls account for up to 20% of acute hospital admissions

Question 8

A 70-year-old woman with severe Parkinson's disease is on co-careldopa and apomorphine. She complains of nausea and vomiting due to her tablets. Which one of the following drugs should be prescribed for these symptoms?

A domperidone

B metoclopramide

C prochlorperazine

D entacapone

E betahistine

Question 9

A 78-year-old woman is greatly distressed by urge incontinence. Which of the following drugs that might be used to treat her is least likely to cause the side effect of a dry mouth?

A oxybutynin

B tolterodine

C imipramine

D desmopressin acetate (DDAVP)

E flavoxate

Question 10

An 82-year-old woman has recently become incontinent of urine. She is constantly dribbling and feels that her bladder is never empty. What type of incontinence is she most likely to have?

A stress incontinence

B urge incontinence

C overflow incontinence

D functional incontinence

E mixed type incontinence

Question 11

A 74-year-old man is admitted to hospital in a dishevelled state with 'failure to cope at home'. At the ward multidisciplinary meeting the physiotherapist states that his Barthel Index is 12. Assessment of which of the following does NOT form part of the Barthel Index score?

A feeding

B bathing
C grooming
D reading
E stairs

Question 12

An 87-year-old woman is admitted to hospital with fever and confusion. She does not give a coherent history and at an early stage you decide to perform an Abbreviated Mental Test Score (AMT) to screen for impaired cognition. Which of the following is NOT a question that forms part of the AMT?

A how old are you?
B what is the time?
C what year is it?
D what were the years of the First World War?
E name of the present prime minister?

Question 13

A 70-year-old man is referred for increasing forgetfulness. On closer questioning, he admits to some urinary incontinence and unsteadiness on walking. He smokes 40 cigarettes a day and has been a heavy drinker in the past. What is most likely diagnosis?

A alcoholic cerebellar degeneration
B Alzheimer's disease

C frontotemporal dementia
D multi-infarct dementia
E normal pressure hydrocephalus

Question 14

An 84-year-old man presents with a 6-month history of increasing confusion, visual hallucinations, reduced mobility and falls. Which type of dementia fits this history best?

A Alzheimer's disease
B Pick's disease
C dementia with Lewy bodies
D Parkinson's disease
E vascular dementia

Question 15

An 82-year-old man is admitted following a fall. The physiotherapist thinks he looks Parkinsonian and asks for your opinion. Which of the following is most supportive of a diagnosis of Parkinson's disease?

A his tremor is most disabling when he is drinking his tea
B his neck is extended and he has a surprised expression, despite paucity of facial movement
C the tremor is worse in his left arm and leg
D you elicit a positive glabellar tap
E you notice marked oro-facial dyskinesia

Answers to Self-assessment

Pain Relief and Palliative Care

A stat dose of either midazolam or levomepromazine will allow you to calculate the 24-hour dose needed for the syringe driver.

Answer to Question 1

B, J

The clinical picture suggests she has developed bowel obstruction. A plain abdominal radiograph would be likely to demonstrate this and also help exclude constipation as a cause. Oral medication is not likely to be absorbed because she is vomiting, hence the recommendation that it be given via a syringe driver. Metoclopramide is a prokinetic agent and can make intestinal colic worse: cyclizine is the antiemetic of first choice.

Avoid a nasogastric tube if possible, but it may give symptomatic relief if vomiting is profuse. Hyoscine butylbromide will help abdominal colic but should be given subcutaneously. Carcinoma of the ovary can cause multiple sites of obstruction: surgery is unlikely to be appropriate in this case, and calling a surgeon is not one of the first two things to do.

Answer to Question 2

B, G

Titrating opioids and adding in co-analgesic drugs for neuropathic pain are the manoeuvres most likely to produce initial improvement in her pain. Intrathecal infusions for neuropathic pain should be tried if standard treatment fails. Further oncological management (radio or chemotherapy) is unlikely to benefit the patient in the short term. Topical treatments (fentanyl patch) are best used when pain is stable because of the long dosing intervals. Parenteral approaches (syringe driver) are unlikely to offer better analgesia if the patient is able to absorb oral medicines. Bisphosphonates and paracetamol are appropriate approaches for bone pain rather than neuropathic pain.

Answer to Question 3

A, H

The woman has intestinal obstruction and requires analgesia as opposed to sedation. Diamorphine prn will allow you to calculate how much extra diamorphine needs to be added to the syringe driver. Hyoscine butylbromide is an antispasmodic and will reduce abdominal colic. A nasogastric tube may help, particularly if there is persistent vomiting, but should be avoided if possible. Further investigation of the obstruction would only be appropriate if the patient were fit enough for surgery, and not before an attempt had been made to control symptoms.

Answer to Question 4

F, I

The patient requires sedation rather than more analgesia.

Answer to Question 5

A, D

Symptoms of opioid withdrawal are often likened to 'cold turkey' i.e. shivering, sweating, lacrimation and rhinorrhea. Patients feel generally unwell and 'fluey' with muscle aches, nausea and vomiting and diarrhoea.

Answer to Question 6

E

Loss of sphincter control can result in faecal incontinence, which is distressing for patients. High dose stimulant laxatives are likely to result in increased faecal incontinence, and co-danthramer can cause rashes if in contact with skin for prolonged periods. A common compromise is to clear the rectum (with manual evacuation or enema), then use low dose laxatives to soften the stool. By using regular enemas, the patient has a predictable bowel movement and a reduced risk of incontinence.

Answer to Question 7

D

160 mg oxycodone over 24 hours is equivalent to 320 mg morphine which is equivalent to approx 106 mg diamorphine.

Answer to Question 8

E

In this circumstance it is best to anticipate problems and avoid the development of pain. A syringe driver with the correct dose of diamorphine and 1/6 dose as breakthrough medication is correct.

Answer to Question 9

D

Hyoscine, cyclizine and levomepromazine have significant antimuscarinic effects that reduce colonic peristalsis and cause constipation. All 5HT3 antagonists (including ondansetron) cause constipation by inhibiting large bowel transit by blocking cholinergic mechanisms. Haloperidol is a dopamine antagonist and not commonly associated with constipation.

Answer to Question 10

D

The history suggests that there may be a neuromuscular cause for his symptoms. Another possibility is external compression, but the endoscopy did not show this. Metoclopramide is both an antidopaminergic and a gastrokinetic agent that may improve oesophageal motility.

Answer to Question 11

E

Hypercalcaemia may well cause these symptoms and should always be checked unless a patient is clearly dying. Another possible metabolic cause of this presentation is renal failure. Opiates rarely cause confusion in the absence of renal failure or overdose for other reasons.

Answer to Question 12

C

Patients with relapsed ovarian cancer do not infrequently develop renal obstruction due to pelvic recurrence. If they are on morphine they may get accumulation of this drug and signs of opioid toxicity superimposed on the signs of renal failure.

Answer to Question 13

A

Bulk forming drugs such as fybogel have little to offer in opioid-induced constipation. Senna can cause abdominal cramps. Co-danthramer can cause skin burns in faecal incontinence: this patient is frail and may not be able to clean herself well and is therefore at risk of this most unpleasant complication. Lactulose can cause bowel distension and increased abdominal cramps.

Answer to Question 14

E

The dose of diamorphine should be 1/3 of the total 24-hour dose of morphine. The prn dose should be 1/6 of the 24 hour dose of diamorphine.

Answer to Question 15

D

Fentanyl Conversion Table

Oral 24 hour morphine dose	Fentanyl dose (μg/hr)
Less than 135 mg	25
135–224	50
225–314	75
315–404	100
405–494	125

Medicine for the Elderly

Answer to Question 1

D

The liver is enlarged, there are several metastases in it (darker areas at right lateral border and anteriorly), and there is ascites (fluid around the liver, appearing black).

With this clinical history the most likely diagnosis is metastatic colonic carcinoma, but other malignancies that are common in this age group (breast, lung, ovary) should be considered.

Answer to Question 2

E

Her symptoms are compatible with anaemia, and the picture shows glossitis and angular cheilosis. Given the history it is likely that she will have poor diet. Deficiency of iron and/or folate is likely in this context and could explain both anaemia and the appearances shown.

Answer to Question 3

G, I

Benzhexol is an anticholinergic drug with the usual anticholinergic side effects: it is said to be more effective for tremor than other features of Parkinson's. Long-term anticholinergic treatment should not be stopped abruptly as patients can deteriorate significantly. Benzhexol should be avoided in patients with dementia due to its neuro-psychiatric side effect profile.

Levodopa combined with a peripheral decarboxylase inhibitor does not cross the blood brain barrier. It can cause motor fluctuations and dyskinesia, and it may discolour urine and sweat.

Amantadine can cause confusion. Apomorphine is a D1 and D2 receptor agonist. Selegiline is a selective inhibitor of monoamine oxidase type B.

Answer to Question 4

C, F

Rigidity is usually present in Parkinson's disease, but not always, and tremor is absent in 30% of cases. Upper body akinesia must be present to diagnose Parkinson's disease. Cumulative lifetime risk of developing Parkinsonism is estimated at 1 in 40. The diagnosis of Parkinson's disease is entirely clinical. Essential tremor and arteriosclerotic pseudo-parkinsonism are commonly misdiagnosed as Parkinson's disease. In essential tremor there may be secondary cogwheeling but no lead pipe rigidity or true akinesia. Rapid progression would suggest non-idiopathic Parkinsonism.

Answer to Question 5

D

A pressure sore/ulcer develops when persistent pressure on a bony site (e.g. heel, greater trochanter) obstructs capillary blood flow: necrosis of tissue can develop within two hours or less. Early stages include changes in skin temperature (warmth or coolness), altered tissue consistency (boggy or firm), and itching. Later stages include partial or full thickness skin loss and destruction of adjacent tissue. Many predisposing factors have been identified (e.g. sepsis, urinary incontinence, diabetes mellitus, immobility) and there are a range of well-validated tools to identify patients at risk.

The use of support surfaces to redistribute pressure has been shown to improve outcomes and reduce costs. Repositioning the patient at least every two hours is also an important component of prevention/management. Attention to nutrition is important to increase wound healing, particularly in those with protein malnutrition.

Answer to Question 6

D

Many psychiatric drugs should not be stopped precipitously, including selective serotonin reuptake inhibitors (SSRIs) such as paroxetine and benzodiazepines (such as lorazepam). If the dose of these medications needs to be changed, this must be done very slowly, otherwise they can produce an acute withdrawal state with worsening confusion and agitation. The same applies to alcohol. Her family can bring in her usual tipple, so that the nurses can monitor intake, otherwise prescribe chlordiazepoxide in reducing doses.

It is important to check her thyroid-stimulating hormone (TSH) level to ensure she is on the correct dose of thyroxine, but this is unlikely to be the cause of the confusion.

Cimetidine can cause confusion in older people and can safely be stopped. Does she still need ulcer-healing treatment? If so, consider a proton pump inhibitor.

Answer to Question 7

C

Tapering and discontinuation of psychotropic drugs, including benzodiazepines and antidepressants, has been shown to reduce the incidence of falls. Some older people with postural hypotension are asymptomatic. Falls account for 6% of acute hospital admissions.

Reducing the number of medications to 4 or less has been shown to reduce the number of falls in older people.

Answer to Question 8

A

Drugs such as apomorphine and bromocriptine cause vomiting through peripheral stimulation of the chemoreceptor trigger zone. Worsening of Parkinson's disease may result from the use of dopamine antagonists: domperidone is much less likely to cross the blood–brain barrier and is therefore the preferred agent in this case. Entacapone is a catechol-O-methyltransferase (COMT) inhibitor which increases levodopa levels, thus worsening nausea and vomiting. Betahistine is used in vertigo.

Answer to Question 9

D

Incontinence should be managed by institution of simple measures such as regular toileting, bladder re-training (gradually increasing the time between voidings), limitation of fluid intake (typically to 1.5 L/day), treatment of atrophic vaginitis, avoidance of bladder irritants (caffeine, alcohol), improving mobility and access to toilets, and sensible choice of clothing.

If these measures fail to provide relief, then pharmacological treatment is appropriate and all of those listed can be effective in urge incontinence. Oxybutinin, tolterodine and flavoxate are all anticholinergics, and imipramine has anticholinergic action, hence all of these are likely to cause a dry mouth.

Answer to Question 10

C

Stress incontinence describes the involuntary leaking of small amounts of urine on coughing, laughing or exercising. Urge incontinence describes an overwhelming and instant urge to pass urine with involuntary emptying of the bladder. Mixed type incontinence has features of both stress and urge incontinence. Functional incontinence describes the situation where the patient is unable to get to the toilet, perhaps secondary to reduced mobility or confusion.

Answer to Question 11

D

The Barthel Index quantitates performance of basic activities of daily living. Ten activities are assessed: feeding, bathing, grooming, dressing, bowels, bladder, toilet, bed/chair, ambulation, stairs. The maximum score is 20.

Answer to Question 12

E

The Abbreviated Mental Test Score (AMT) asks the following ten questions:
- Age
- Time (to nearest hour)
- Address for recall at the end (e.g. 42 West Street)
- What year is it?
- Name of institution
- Recognition of two persons (e.g. nurse and doctor)
- Date of birth (day and month)
- Year of First World War
- Name of present monarch
- Count backwards from 20 to 1

Answer to Question 13

E

The triad of dementia, urinary incontinence and gait disturbance is classically associated with normal pressure hydrocephalus.

Answer to Question 14

C

There is some overlap between the different types of dementia, but in this case there are clues that this is dementia with Lewy bodies (DLB) with the early development of instability, falls and hallucinations. Other features include fluctuating cognition, depression and delusions.

Treatment is usually symptomatic, but remember that neuroleptic drugs such as haloperidol will worsen Parkinsonian features, so consider using atypical antipsychotic agents such as quetiapine. There is some evidence that the dementia may respond to anticholinesterase inhibitors.

Dementia associated with Parkinson's disease tends to occur much later in the course of the disease.

Answer to Question 15

C

Parkinson's disease is typically asymmetrical at presentation. The tremor is typically a rest tremor so it is usually possible for the patient to drink (unlike benign essential tremor, where action such as drinking a cup of tea makes the tremor worse). Marked chewing movements and lip-smacking suggest drug-induced Parkinsonism and an extended neck and raised eyebrows suggest progressive supranuclear palsy; the neck is characteristically flexed in Parkinson's disease. A positive glabeller tap is common in normal older people and is falling out of favour as a diagnostic sign in younger patients too.

The Medical Masterclass series

Clinical Skills

General Clinical Issues

Pain Relief and Palliative Care

Medicine for the Elderly

Emergency Medicine

Infectious Diseases and Dermatology

Infectious Diseases

Cardiology and Respiratory Medicine

Cardiology

Respiratory Medicine

Gastroenterology and Hepatology

Neurology, Ophthalmology and Psychiatry

Neurology

Nephrology

Rheumatology and Clinical Immunology

Index